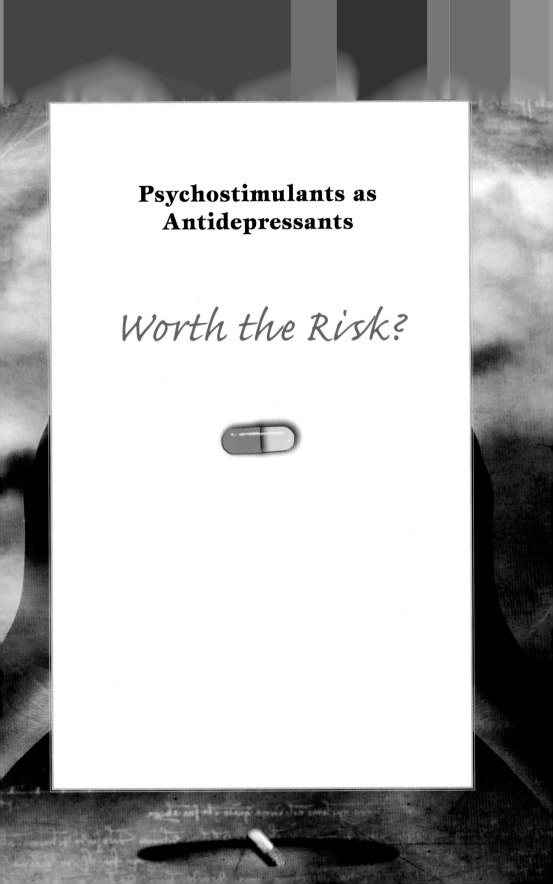

Psychostimulants as Antidepressants

Worth the Risk?

ANTIDEPRESSANTS

ANTIDEPRESSANTS

Psychostimulants as Antidepressants

Worth the Risk?

by Craig Russell

Mason Crest Publishers

Philadelphia

Mason Crest Publishers Inc.
370 Reed Road
Broomall, Pennsylvania 19008
(866) MCP-BOOK (toll free)

First printing
1 2 3 4 5 6 7 8 9 10
Library of Congress Cataloging-in-Publication Data

Russell, Craig, 1952–
  Psychostimulants as antidepressants : worth the risk? / by Craig
Russell.
    p. cm. — (Antidepressants)
  Includes bibliographical references and index.
  ISBN 1-4222-0107-4   ISBN (series) 1-4222-0094-9
  1. Stimulants—Juvenile literature. 2. Psychotropic drugs—Juvenile lit-
erature. 3. Antidepressants—Juvenile literature. I. Title. II. Series.
  RM332.R875 2007
  615'.788—dc22
                          2006011807

Interior design by MK Bassett-Harvey.
Interiors produced by Harding House Publishing Service, Inc.
www.hardinghousepages.com.
Cover design by Peter Culatta.
Printed in the Hashemite Kingdom of Jordan.

This book is meant to educate and should not be used as an alternative to appropriate medical care. Its creators have made every effort to ensure that the information presented is accurate—but it is not intended to substitute for the help and
services of trained professionals.

Contents

Introduction

by Andrew M. Kleiman, M.D.

From ancient Greece through the twenty-first century, the experience of sadness and depression is one of the many that define humanity. As long as human beings have felt emotions, they have endured depression. Experienced by people from every race, socioeconomic class, age group, and culture, depression is an emotional and physical experience that millions of people suffer each day. Despite being described in literature and music; examined by countless scientists, philosophers, and thinkers; and studied and treated for centuries, depression continues to remain as complex and mysterious as ever.

In today's Western culture, hearing about depression and treatments for depression is common. Adolescents in particular are bombarded with information, warnings, recommendations, and suggestions. It is critical that adolescents and young people have an understanding of depression and its impact on an individual's psychological and physical health, as well as the treatment options available to help those who suffer from depression.

Why? Because depression can lead to poor school performance, isolation from family and friends, alcohol and drug abuse, and even suicide. This doesn't have to be the case, since many useful and promising treatments exist to relieve the suffering of those with depression. Treatments for depression may also pose certain risks, however.

Since the beginning of civilization, people have been trying to alleviate the suffering of those with depression. Modern-day medicine and psychology have taken the understanding and treatment of depression to new heights. Despite their shortcomings, these treatments have helped millions and millions of people lead happier, more fulfilling and prosperous lives that would not be possible in generations past. These treatments, however, have their own risks, and for some people, may not be effective at all. Much work in neuroscience, medicine, and psychology needs to be done in the years to come.

Many adolescents experience depression, and this book series will help young people to recognize depression both in themselves and in those around them. It will give them the basic understanding of the history of depression and the various treatments that have been used to combat depression over the years. The books will also provide a basic scientific understanding of depression, and the many biological, psychological, and alternative treatments available to someone suffering from depression today.

Each person's brain and biology, life experiences, thoughts, and day-to-day situations are unique. Similarly, each individual experiences depression and sadness in a unique way. Each adolescent suffering from depression thus requires a distinct, individual treatment plan that best suits his or her needs. This series promises to be a vital resource for helping young people recognize and understand depression, and make informed and thoughtful decisions regarding treatment.

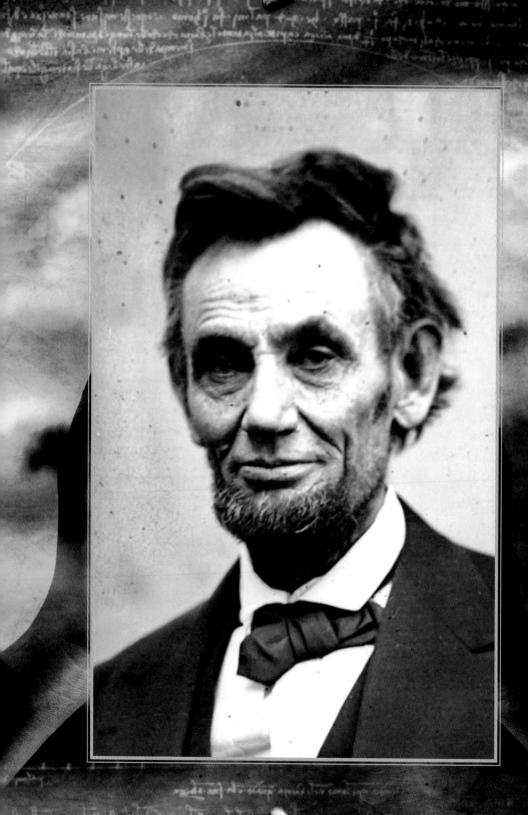

Chapter 1

What Is Depression?

On February 27, 1860, Abraham Lincoln's life would change forever—and when it did, he didn't seem to care.

His debates with Stephen Douglas in 1858 had earned him some notice, and he had been invited to speak in New York City. So many people wanted to hear him that the location was moved to the Great Hall at Cooper Union, which held almost fifteen hundred people. This was the biggest opportunity of his career, and he was very worried about it. A friend said Lincoln had "a woe-begone look on his face," and Lincoln confessed to him that he was afraid he had made a mistake in coming to New York.

When he finished speaking, however, the spellbound audience "erupted in thunderous applause." One person said,

"When I came out of the hall, my face glowing with excitement and my frame all aquiver, a friend, with his eyes aglow, asked me what I thought of Abe Lincoln. . . . I said 'He's the greatest man since St. Paul.'" Lincoln had taken a giant step toward becoming president of the United States. The next day's *New York Tribune* reported that "no man ever before made such an impression on his first appeal to a New York audience."

Afterward, however, Lincoln seemed unaffected by either the praise or the applause. Charles Nott, who walked back to Lincoln's hotel with him, said that Lincoln seemed to be a "sad and lonely man."

Later that year, Lincoln attended the Illinois state Republican convention. When he walked to the stage, "the crowd roared in approval. Men threw hats and canes into the air, shaking the hall so much that the awning over the stage collapsed; according to an early account, 'the roof was literally cheered off the building.'" And yet many in the crowd could sense that Lincoln did not seem triumphant—or even pleased. One person said, "I then thought him one of the most ***diffident*** and worst plagued men I ever saw." The next day, the lieutenant governor of Illinois noticed Lincoln sitting alone at the end of the hall with his head in his hands. As he approached him, Lincoln looked up and said, "I'm not very well."

His friends called him "***melancholy***." He would often cry in public, or tell jokes and stories at inappropriate times—he needed the laughs, he said, in order to survive. When he was young, he spoke of suicide; when he was older, he said that he saw life as hard and grim and full of misery. A friend of his said that "no element of Mr. Lincoln's character was so marked, obvious and ingrained as his mysterious and profound melancholy." And his former law partner said, "His melancholy dripped from him as he walked."

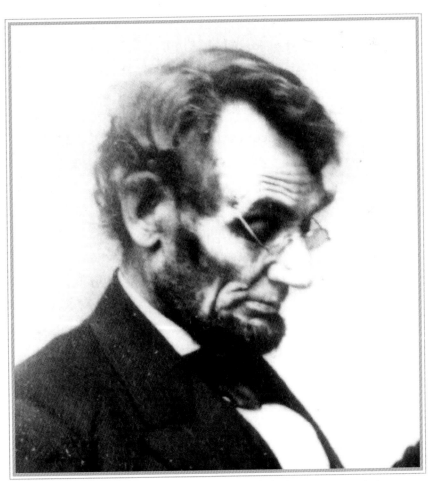

Abraham Lincoln went through life immersed deep in depression—and yet his influence on America has endured for more than a hundred years.

Melancholy

Before modern technology changed our view of medicine, melancholy was *one of the "four* humors." *A humor was a temperament, or a disposition. Doctors used to think that there were four basic personality types, each based on four fluids found in the human body. People who were generally happy, popular, and fun-loving had lots of blood and were called* sanguine. *Calm, unemotional people had lots of* phlegm *in them and were called* phlegmatic. *People who got angry easily and had a bad temper had lots of* yellow bile *and were called* choleric, *while those who were irritable and despondent had too much* black bile *in them and were called* melancholic.

Today, many psychiatrists would say that Lincoln, like millions of other Americans, suffered from depression. Almost 10 percent of Americans, or about twenty million people, suffer from some form of depression every year, and as many as one-quarter of the population will become depressed at some point in their lives. Women are twice as likely as men to experience depression.

The *American Heritage Dictionary* defines depression as "a psychiatric disorder characterized by an inability to concentrate, insomnia, loss of appetite, **anhedonia**, feelings of extreme sadness, guilt, helplessness and hopelessness, and thoughts of death." The authors of *Caring for Depression* say that depression "consists of feelings of sadness or **apathy** accompanied by symptoms such as irritability, poor concentration, diminished or increased appetite, or loss of interest in activities usually enjoyed."

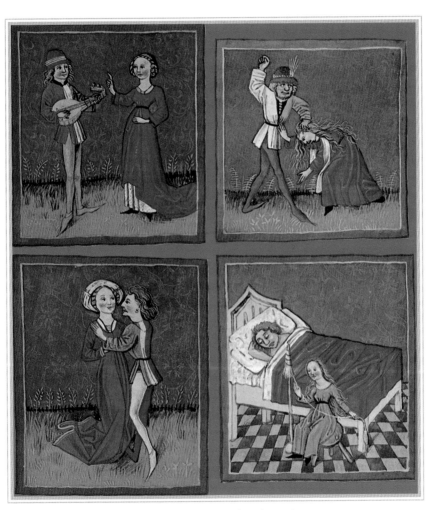

A medieval portrayal of the four humors: top, left: melancholic; top, right: choleric; bottom left: sanguine; bottom right: phlegmatic.

The *Diagnostic and Statistical Manual* of the American Psychiatric Society (DSM) lists nine symptoms of depression:

1. depressed mood
2. diminished interest or pleasure in activities
3. weight gain or loss or change in appetite
4. insomnia or hypersomnia (excessive sleep)
5. ***psychomotor agitation*** or retardation (slowing down)
6. fatigue or loss of energy
7. feelings of worthlessness or excessive or inappropriate guilt
8. diminished ability to think or concentrate or indecisiveness
9. recurrent thoughts of death or suicidal ***ideation*** or suicide attempt

People who have five of these nine symptoms for two weeks or longer, according to the DSM, have a "depressive disorder."

Besides Abraham Lincoln, such people as Michelangelo, Isaac Newton, Ludwig von Beethoven, Mark Twain, Emily Dickinson, and Winston Churchill are said to have suffered from depression. In our own time, depression has struck Barbara Bush, Drew Barrymore, Kurt Cobain, and Winona Ryder (among many others).

The Varieties of Mood Disorders

There are various forms of mood disorders. The three most common are major depression, dysthymia, and bipolar disor-

History of Depression

Depression is certainly not a new problem. Hippocrates wrote about it in the fifth century B.C.E. and provided the first known definition of depression as a specific disorder. "If fear or distress last for a long time," he wrote, "it is melancholia." A hundred years later, Aristotle wrote that "we are often in the condition of feeling grief without being able to ascribe any cause to it; such feelings occur to a slight degree in everyone, but those who are thoroughly possessed by them acquire them as a permanent part of their nature." In his 1621 book The Anatomy of Melancholy, *Robert Burton defined depression as "a kind of dotage without a fever, having for his ordinary companions fear and sadness, without any apparent occasion."*

der, which is also called manic-depressive illness. Major depression is the most common of the three, affecting almost ten million people, or 5 percent of the population, every year. About 75 percent of those who experience an episode of major depression will experience another one at some point in their lives.

Major Depression

People experiencing major depression feel sad all the time and no longer enjoy things that once made them happy. Often

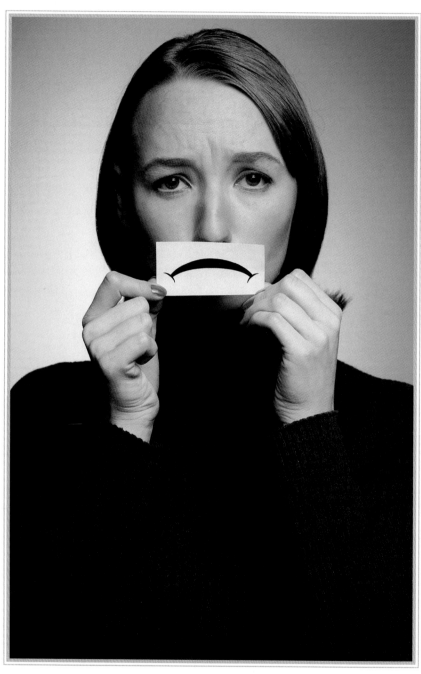

A major depression makes an individual feel sad all the time, regardless of circumstances.

they have trouble sleeping, can't concentrate well, and lose their appetite. They might feel guilty about things and think of killing themselves. They tend to feel worthless, hopeless, and unable to do anything to stop these feelings. Major depression, which is also known as clinical depression, unipolar depression, or major depressive disorder, usually occurs between the ages of twenty-five and forty-four, though it can occur at any time in a person's life. This disorder usually presents in men earlier than in women, but over the course of a lifetime, it is more common in women.

Dysthymia

Dysthymia is similar to major depression, but the symptoms are milder and last longer. Some of these symptoms are poor performance at school or at work, shyness and withdrawal from social situations, conflicts with family members, and sleeplessness. People with dysthymia aren't as disabled as those with major depression, but they don't function or feel very well, either. About 3 percent of Americans will experience dysthymia at some time in their lives. Like major depression, dysthymia occurs twice as often in women as in men. Also, it is more common among poor people and unmarried people. While the symptoms of dysthymia usually appear when people are teenagers or in early adulthood, they may not emerge until middle age. When a person with dysthymia then falls into a more severe major depression, it is described as a "double depression."

Bipolar Disorder

The third common type of mood disorder is called bipolar disorder. Like dysthymia, bipolar disorder usually develops during the teenage or early adult years, though it may emerge at any time in a person's life. People with this form of depression experience dramatic mood swings.

When people with this disorder are manic, they're very energetic, active, and restless. Their thoughts race, and they jump quickly from one idea to the next. They're unable to concentrate and find that they don't seem to need much sleep. Sometimes their judgment becomes poor, and they go on spending sprees. They might become aggressive and **provocative** and deny that anything is wrong.

When their mood swings the other way and they become depressed, they feel sad, anxious, or empty. They're restless, have little energy, and they find it difficult to remember things or make decisions. Often they feel worthless, helpless, and guilty, and they think about suicide. Sometimes, when these episodes of mania or depression are severe, they might **hallucinate** or become **delusional**. For example, during a manic state, a person might begin to believe that he's president of the United States or has great wealth and power. During a depressed state, this same person might believe he's committed a terrible crime or that his life is totally ruined.

Treating Depression

For much of human history, no help was available for those with depression. People like Abraham Lincoln had to learn on their own how to cope with their situation as best they could. But with the rise of psychiatry during the twentieth century, people began taking a different view of depression. Today, doctors can use a variety of techniques to treat all types of depression. Sometimes they find that counseling sessions alone work best to help people cope with their depression. Other times, though, they find that their patients need more than just counseling. Sometimes they find that their patients need medications.

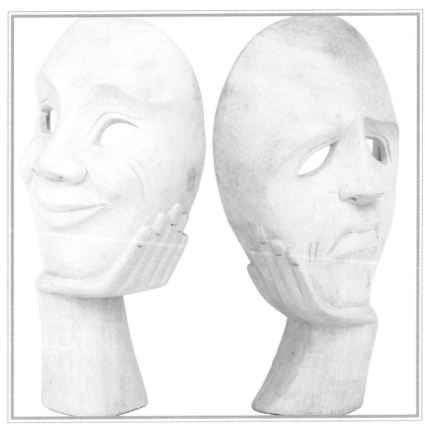

Individuals with bipolar disorder experience mood swings between extreme happiness and depression.

Usually, depression is treated with drugs called antidepressants. The first antidepressant, iproniazid, was discovered by accident in the 1950s. It was originally developed as a treatment for tuberculosis. But when doctors found that it not only helped patients' tuberculosis, it also improved their mood and stimulated activity, they began prescribing it for people with clinical depression. During its first year, about 400,000 people were treated with it. The second type of antidepressants, called tricyclics, was also discovered by accident.

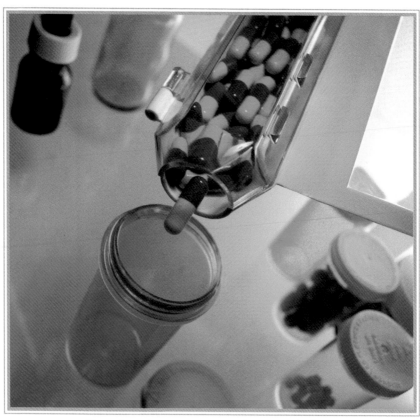

Medication has proven to be one of the most effective ways to treat depression.

Brand Name vs. Generic Name

Talking about psychiatric drugs can be confusing, because every drug has at least two names: its "generic name" and the "brand name" that the pharmaceutical company uses to market the drug. Generic names come from the drugs' chemical structure, while drug companies use brand names in order to inspire public recognition and loyalty for their products.

Here are the brand names and generic names for some common psychiatric drugs:

Elavil®	*amitriptyline hydrochloride*
Librium®	*chlorodiazepoxide*
Marplan®	*isocarboxazid*
Nardil®	*phenelzine sulfate*
Norpramin®	*desipramine hydrochloride*
Paxil®	*paroxetine hydrochloride*
Periactin®	*cyproheptadine hydrochloride*
Prozac®	*fluoxetine hyrdrochloride*
Tofranil®	*imipramine hydrochloride*
Valium®	*diazepam*
Xanax®	*alprazolam*
Zofran®	*ondansetron hydrochloride*
Zoloft®	*sertraline hydrochloride*

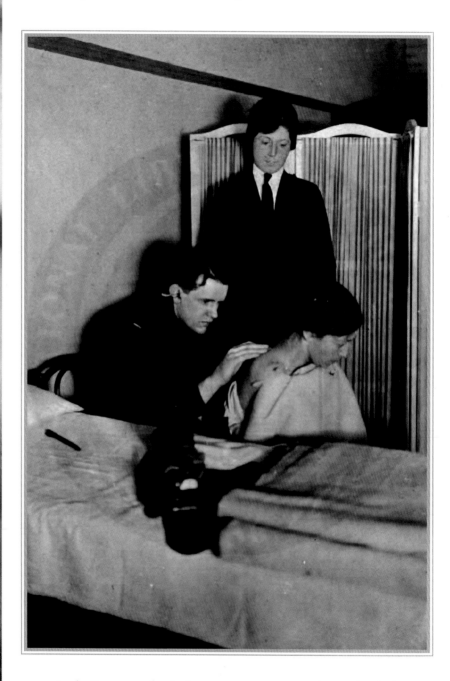

As doctors sought better ways to treat tuberculosis in the first half of the twentieth century, they stumbled across iproniazid, an effective treatment of depression.

Tricyclics were originally developed to treat **schizophrenia**. They failed at that, but doctors again noticed that they improved the mood of the patients who took them.

While iproniazid revolutionized the treatment of depression, people taking it had to follow a strict diet to avoid the drug's dangerous side effects. Tricyclics also elevated the mood of patients with depression and increased their energy levels, but they too had side effects that doctors wished to avoid. However, research into how tricyclics worked helped to develop the newest generation of antidepressants, called selective serotonin reuptake inhibitors, or SSRIs. The first and most widely used SSRI is called Prozac® (fluoxetine). Other common SSRIs include Luvox® (fluvoxamine), Paxil® (paroxetine), and Zoloft® (sertraline). When none of the antidepressant drugs work well enough, however, doctors sometimes try another medication, called a psychostimulant.

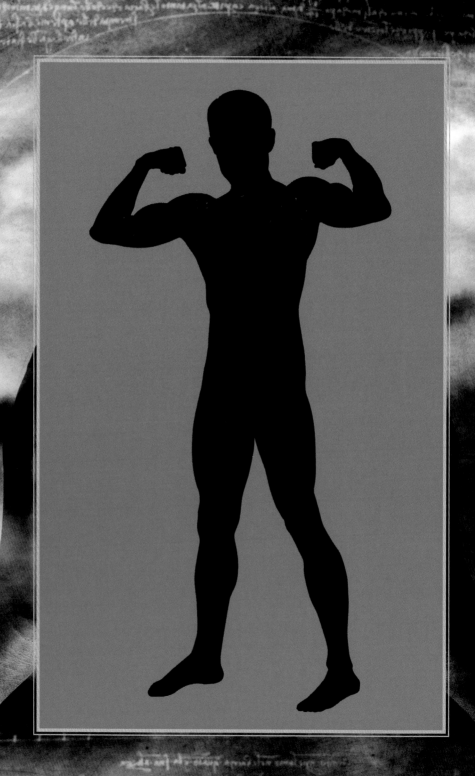

Chapter 2

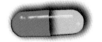

Why Are Psychostimulants Used to Treat Depression?

espite the research and care that went into the creation of SSRIs, they don't always work as well as people would like them to work. For example, it can often take two to three weeks for an antidepressant to have an effect, and sometimes patients can't afford to wait that long. One such situation occurs when the patient is not just clinically depressed but is also physically ill.

Depression and Physical Illness

It's hard to pinpoint just how many physically ill people also suffer from clinical depression. Sometimes, physical diseases can produce symptoms of depression, while at other times they can hide them. One researcher, for instance, found that 5 percent of his cancer patients also had major depression, while another found major depression in 42 percent of his patients. Studies of people with multiple sclerosis found depression in as few as 6 percent and as many as 57 percent. One doctor found major depression in 83 percent of his patients being treated for other diseases.

Depression can have major consequences for those who are also physically ill. It can cause them to lose their appetite

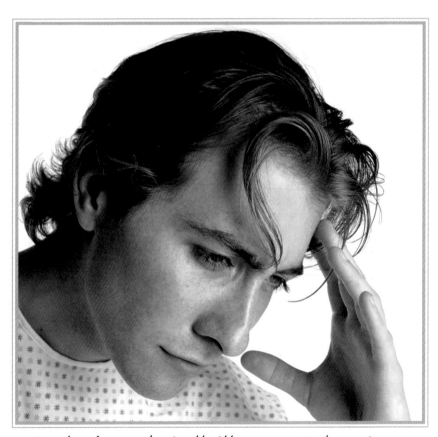

People who are physically ill are prone to depression— and depression can worsen their physical well-being.

and thus weaken their immune system. It can cause surgical wounds to take longer to heal, and it can make individuals unable or unwilling to help take care of themselves. Finally, their negative thoughts make recovery from both their depression and their physical illness more difficult. Under these conditions, it's important that doctors find a way to relieve symptoms of depression as quickly as possible.

Take, for instance, the case of "Dan Johnson." At the age of fifty, he had just received a heart transplant. According to the team of doctors who had performed the transplant, Dan had "lost his will to live." He wouldn't eat, he slept all day, and he would not participate in his own care. This threatened his recovery from this very serious surgery.

Heart Transplant

The first heart transplant took place in 1967. Dr. Christiaan Barnard of Cape Town, South Africa, transplanted the heart of a twenty-five-year-old woman who had died in an automobile accident into the body of Louis Washkansky, a fifty-five-year-old man dying of heart failure. He died eighteen days later. The procedure was rarely performed until antirejection drugs were developed. As of 2001, more than 100,000 heart transplants have been done. Today, 75 percent of heart transplant patients live more than five years with their new hearts.

The doctors asked a psychiatrist to examine Dan, and he prescribed 2.5 milligrams of the psychostimulant Ritalin (methylphenidate) twice a day. At first, it had little effect, so over the next three days they increased his dosage to 10 milligrams twice a day. As a result, his energy level increased. He began talking more, seemed livelier, and started to eat again. Because of this, his physical condition improved, and he was finally able to leave the intensive care unit.

Another instance of using a psychostimulant as an antidepressant concerned a thirty-seven-year-old man named "John Wallace." He had suffered from **congestive heart failure** for three months, and his illness had begun to affect his kidneys as well. Without treatment, the doctors expected him to die in four to six weeks. Despite this, he refused to allow doctors to evaluate him.

Doctors learned that John's wife had recently died and that he had two small children. They also learned that he didn't speak much, and for eight months he had eaten and slept very little. A psychiatrist thought John's refusal to cooperate with his doctors was a result of clinical depression. However, because of John's physical problems, the psychiatrist did not want to prescribe a standard antidepressant. More important, however, they needed something that would act quickly because his health was rapidly getting worse.

The doctors in this case also turned to a psychostimulant. They began giving John 5 milligrams of Dexedrine® (dextro-amphetamine) every morning. Within twenty-four hours, his spirits had improved a great deal. He began talking to the hospital staff and to his family and friends. He also agreed to

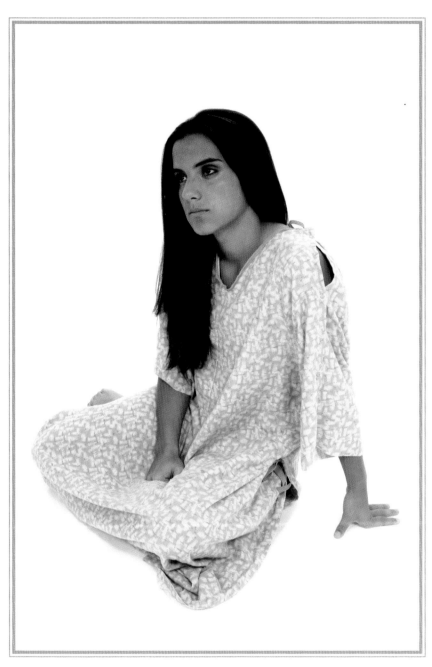

A psychostimulant may be an appropriate treatment for someone who is suffering from both depression and a physical illness.

having a doctor evaluate his medical condition. When that showed that he needed a heart transplant, he agreed to that as well.

Depression and the Elderly

Some doctors are finding that psychostimulants can also be useful in treating depression among the elderly. For example, after sixty-two-year-old Edie Dominquez received a liver transplant, he said he "felt like garbage." His mood and energy were so bad that he couldn't start his physical therapy, and he was having trouble walking. But after his doctor started giving him Ritalin, he quickly became more responsive, more talkative, and began eating better. Thanks to Ritalin, Edie said, "I don't feel depressed."

Depression and the Terminally Ill

In addition, psychostimulants can help treat depression in people who are terminally ill. "Alma Ferrone," for instance, had been diagnosed with breast cancer, which had spread throughout her body. In addition, she had broken two vertebrae in her back and had been hospitalized for a blocked blood vessel in her lungs. The drugs her doctors had been giving her for pain had been doing such a poor job that she could rarely sleep past four in the morning. Her appetite had become poor, and she had lost interest in her hobbies. She told her doctors,

> My future is over. There is nothing good ahead for me. I worry about how much suffering is ahead, about my daughter, and about how my husband will manage. If it weren't for

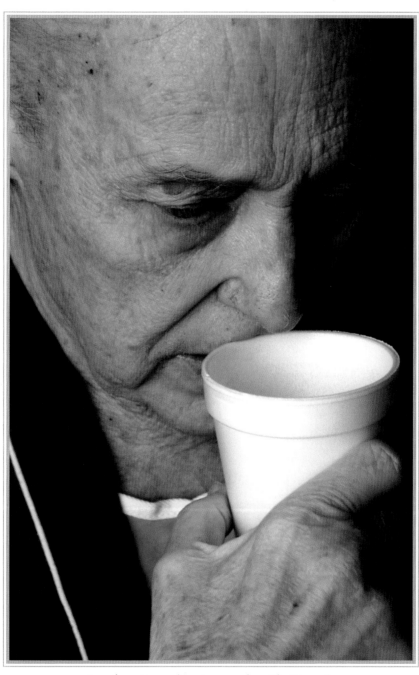

Psychostimulants can be effective for treating depression in the elderly.

my religion, I would call that doctor who kills people. I used to feel proud of being a good mother and wife. But I've lost that. All I can see is how much suffering I am putting people through. I can't forgive myself for that.

When the doctors increased her pain medicine, her mood improved slightly, but the symptoms of depression remained. However, antidepressants can take weeks to take effect, and they believed Ms. Ferrone had at most a few months left to live. As a result, her doctors decided to give her psychostimulants instead. Because psychostimulants act much more quickly

Hospice

The word "hospice" comes from the Latin word "hospitum," or "guesthouse," from which we also get the words "hospital" and "hospitality." It refers to a program that provides physical care as well as spiritual and emotional support to the dying and their families. The first hospice in the United States was established in New Haven, Connecticut, in 1974. Today, 80 percent of hospice care takes place in the patient's home, a family member's home, or a nursing home. It allows people to die surrounded by friends and family rather than in the often cold and unfriendly environment of a hospital.

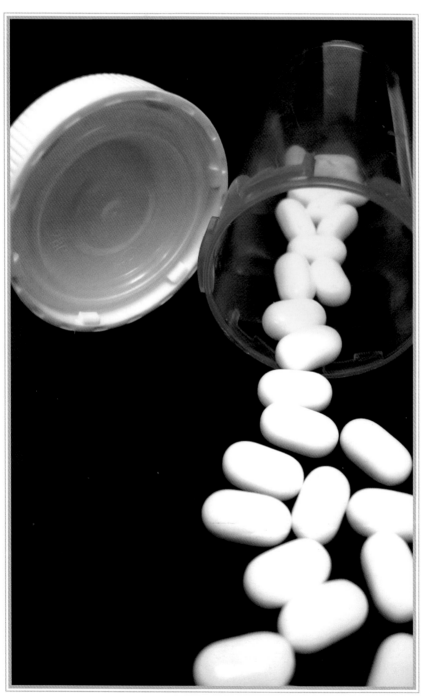

Psychostimulants work more quickly than antidepressants.

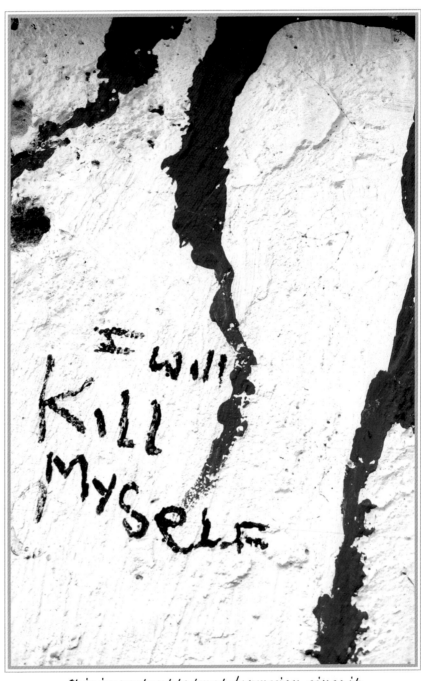

*It is important to treat depression, since it
can be fatal if it leads to suicide.*

than antidepressants, patients who are extremely weakened and tired can often feel their depression start to lift within twenty-four hours.

At first, Ms. Ferrone said that she was "glad to go to God," and she was reluctant to begin taking any drug. Finally, though, she agreed to take 2.5 milligrams of Ritalin twice a day. Within two days, her family said, she had more energy, was sleeping better, and had less pain. After her doctors increased her dosage, she said she was feeling less downhearted and was looking forward to the holidays. Ten days after she began taking Ritalin, her family felt that she had fully recovered from her depression. She was then able to enter a hospice program, where she continued taking Ritalin. Her depression did not return, and after she died, her family said that they were grateful that "she remained herself until the very end."

Treatment-Resistant Depression

Occasionally, a person's depression won't respond to the usual antidepressants. In some of these instances, a doctor might prescribe a psychostimulant. Take "Peter Thompson," for instance. At the age of forty-nine, he had a twenty-nine-year history of treatment-resistant depression. The world often seemed unreal to him. He was anxious around other people and found no pleasure from activities like eating or being with friends. He sometimes thought about killing himself. Over the years, he had tried almost every kind of antidepressant. He had also tried *psychotherapy* and even *electroconvulsive therapy*.

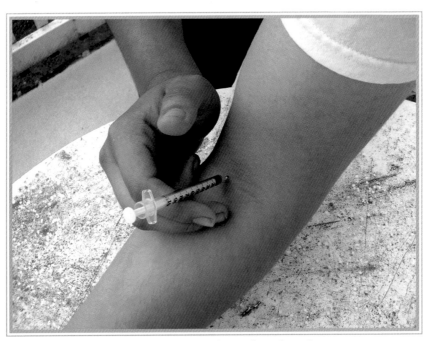

Depression can make it harder for an
individual to battle drug addiction.

He did have a partial response to Parnate® (tranylcypro-
mine) and the antidepressant Wellbutrin® (bupropion), but
his symptoms remained. When his doctors added the psychostimulant Provigil® (modafinil), however, his condition began
to improve significantly. Peter said that adding modafinil gave
him a greater feeling of being connected to things. The drug
made it easier for him to get out of bed in the morning and
start the day. He even began exercising and lost fifteen pounds.
He said that he was "multitudes better with modafinil, and I
would be dead without it."

"Susan Baker" provides another example of a psychostimulant working well to alleviate depression. At the age of

twenty-one, she had a six-year history of various psychiatric illnesses and was also addicted to heroin. Although she did show a partial response to some antidepressants, she was unable to kick her heroin habit. Her "whole life," she said, "was being run by drugs."

However, when her doctors started giving her 200 milligrams of modafinil every morning, she finally began feeling better. Her mood improved, she said, because she was "happy about getting things done." She also said the modafinil helped reduce her desire for heroin. As a result, she was able to find a job and live a relatively stable life.

Antidepressants will help most people with depression feel better. But for some people, in certain situations, psychostimulants can work where antidepressants can't—and in other cases, pyschostimulants can give people the emotional and physical boost they need to allow other treatments to take effect.

Chapter 3

What Is a Psychostimulant?

Not all psychostimulants are prescription drugs. In fact, millions of people around the world begin every day by taking a psychostimulant. Many of them would probably tell you they find it very difficult to get going in the morning without it, and that they become cranky and irritable when they can't have any. The caffeine found in their morning coffee is perhaps the most popular drug in the world. A 2003 survey by the National Coffee Association found that 166.6 million Americans drank coffee. More than half of them drink it every day. People also get caffeine from tea and some soft drinks.

The History of Nicotine

Tobacco, which is the source of the nicotine in cigars and cigarettes, is responsible for the success of the first English colony in North America. The English who established Jamestown, Virginia, in 1607 did very poorly during the first years of its existence—until the Natives showed the settlers how to successfully grow tobacco. Then the settlers were able to make enough money to justify their presence in the New World. In 1618, Virginia farmers sent 50,000 pounds of tobacco to England. Eight years later, that number had increased to 300,000. Without tobacco, the English might never have succeeded, and there might never have been a United States of America. Unfortunately, nicotine has led to a host of other problems for Americans.

Nicotine, found in cigarettes, is another popular psychostimulant. In 2004, the Centers for Disease Control and Prevention estimated that about 21 percent of Americans were current smokers.

The *American Heritage Dictionary* defines a psychostimulant as "a drug having antidepressant or mood-elevating properties." The word comes from "psycho-," which means "mind," and "stimulant," which is a substance that "temporarily arouses or accelerates physiological or organic activity."

Perhaps the most powerful natural psychostimulant is cocaine, which comes from the leaves of the coca plant, found in South America. The natives there would chew coca leaves to give them increased energy. Sigmund Freud, the founder of psychoanalysis, wrote that cocaine was "a magical drug." Cocaine was one of the original ingredients of Coca-Cola, which was marketed at first as a nerve tonic, stimulant, and headache remedy. Cocaine was not made illegal in the United States until 1914.

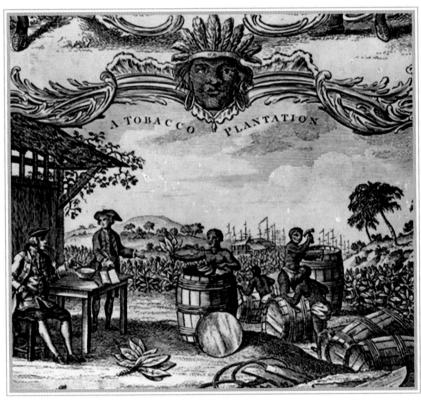

Much of American history centers around a psychostimulant—the nicotine found in tobacco.

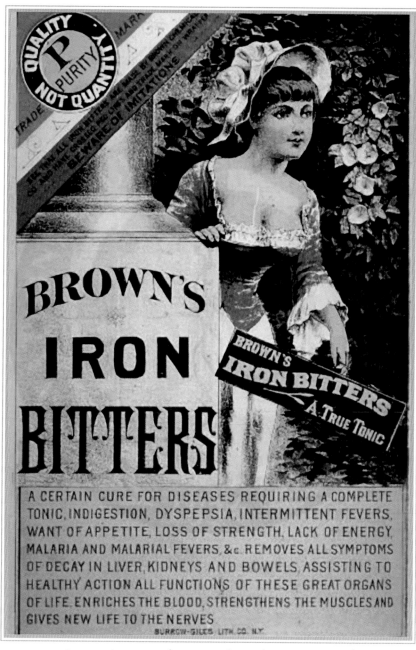

"Iron Bitters," advertised in the nineteenth century as a tonic for nerves and a host of other ailments, were really cocaine.

The History of Amphetamines

Amphetamines were the first **synthetic** psychostimulants. They were created in Germany in 1887. The earliest popular amphetamine product was the Benzedrine Inhaler, which appeared in 1932. It was available without a prescription and helped people with asthma and nasal congestion. In 1935, Dexedrine® (dextroamphetamine) appeared on the market. Dexedrine was superior to Benzedrine because it gave more stimulation to a person's central nervous system, while producing less general nervousness. Another type of amphetamine, Desoxyn® (methamphetamine), was marketed in

Methamphetamines

The Department of Justice calls methamphetamine "by far the most prevalent synthetic controlled substance clandestinely manufactured in the United States today." Stronger than amphetamine and easier to make, it was first synthesized in Japan in 1919. The German military was supplied with millions of methamphetamine tablets during the first half of 1940, near the beginning of World War II. The military leadership believed these drugs would help their soldiers, sailors, and pilots defeat the French. Like other forms of amphetamines, methamphetamine alleviates fatigue and gives the user a feeling of alertness and well-being.

1942. During World War II, amphetamines were widely distributed to soldiers to help keep them awake and alert. After the war, truck drivers began using "uppers," which were then legal, to keep them awake on long hauls. Students took "pep pills" to help them study. Many people used amphetamines to help them lose weight. Both Adolf Hitler and John F. Kennedy are believed to have been heavy users of amphetamines.

Bernard Weiss and Victor Laties studied amphetamines extensively in the early 1960s. They found that amphetamines improved human performance in a number of ways. For example, they made people more aware and accurate when they performed repetitive and boring tasks. They also improved people's attitude toward those tasks. In addition, they discovered that people found amphetamines very pleasurable. In one study, for instance, they injected volunteers with heroin, morphine, amphetamines, and a *placebo*. None of the volunteers knew what they were being injected with. When asked which was the most pleasurable, they overwhelmingly chose amphetamines.

Because people often find them pleasurable, amphetamines can be very addictive. In many human and animal studies from the 1930s to the present, researchers found that if given the chance, subjects will continue to take amphetamines. Laboratory rats, for instance, will repeatedly choose amphetamines—and Ritalin—over food and starve to death rather than give up their drug. Researchers also found that as time went on, people needed more and more of the drug to attain the same feeling.

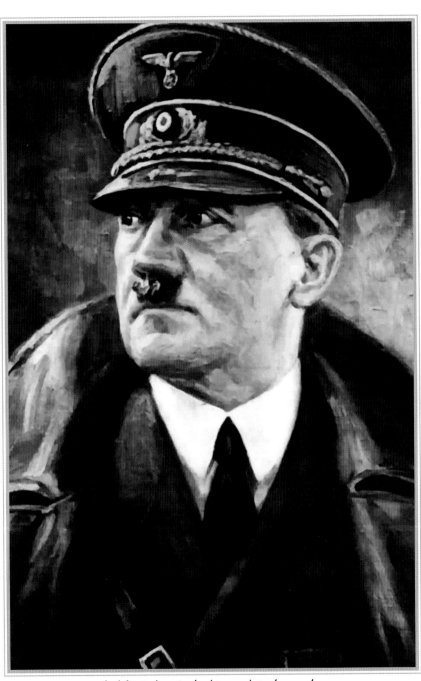

Adolf Hitler is believed to have been addicted to amphetamines.

Varieties of Psychostimulants

Methylphenidate was synthesized in 1944 and introduced into the United States in 1955, an unsuccessful attempt to create a stimulant that was not addictive. Its chemical structure is similar to amphetamine and has similar effects. While

Drug Approval

Before a drug can be marketed in the United States, it must be officially approved by the Food and Drug Administration (FDA). Today's FDA is the primary consumer protection agency in the United States. Operating under the authority given it by the government and guided by laws established throughout the twentieth century, the FDA has established a rigorous drug approval process that verifies the safety, effectiveness, and accuracy of labeling for any drug marketed in the United States.

While the United States has the FDA for the approval and regulation of drugs and medical devices, Canada has a similar organization called the Therapeutic Product Directorate (TPD). The TPD is a division of Health Canada, the Canadian government department of health. The TPD regulates drugs, medical devises, disinfectants, and sanitizers with disinfectant claims. Some of the things that the TPD monitors are quality, effectiveness, and safety. Just as the FDA must approve new drugs in the United States, the TPD must approve new drugs in Canada before those drugs can enter the market.

it is perhaps most recognizable under the brand name Ritalin, it is also sold, in slightly different formulations, under the brand names Focalin®, Concerta®, Metadate®, Methylin®, and Rubifen®.

Pemoline, which is marketed as Cylert®, came on the market in 1975 (and was withdrawn in 2005). Pemoline is the only psychostimulant with a basic chemical structure different than the amphetamines or methylphenidate.

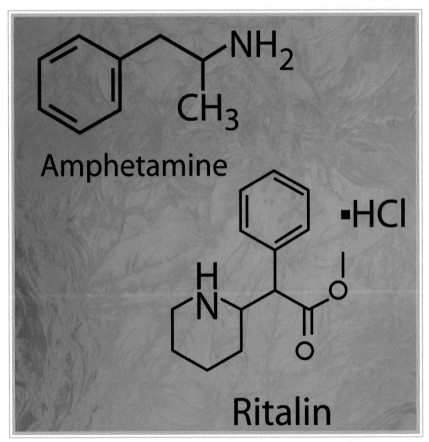

The chemical structure of Ritalin is similar to amphetamine—and it affects the body in similar ways.

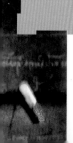

Adderall was first sold in the 1960s as an aid to weight loss. Since 1995, this combination of amphetamine and dextroamphetamine has quickly become one of the most popular drugs in the United States.

Modafinil (Provigil) was developed in France in 1981 specifically to treat depression and was approved by the U.S. Food and Drug Administration (FDA) in 1998. As with amphetamines and pemoline, no one is sure exactly how modafinil works. It appears, however, to work differently than either of those drugs. Instead of stimulating the central nervous system, it apparently affects the hypothalamus, the part of the brain thought to be responsible for wakefulness.

Who Needs Stimulation?

The Federal Drug Control Amendment of 1965 gave the FDA greater control over amphetamines and other psychostimulants. Today, they are legally available only by prescription. Their main legal use is for the treatment of attention-deficit hyperactive disorder (ADHD). They are also often prescribed for treatment of narcolepsy, a disorder that affects more than 100,000 Americans. People with narcolepsy experience sudden and often uncontrollable attacks of deep sleep. It appears to be a hereditary disorder that not only affects humans but also animals like cats, dogs, horses, and even Brahma bulls. The stimulation that drugs like Provigil provide helps to keep people awake.

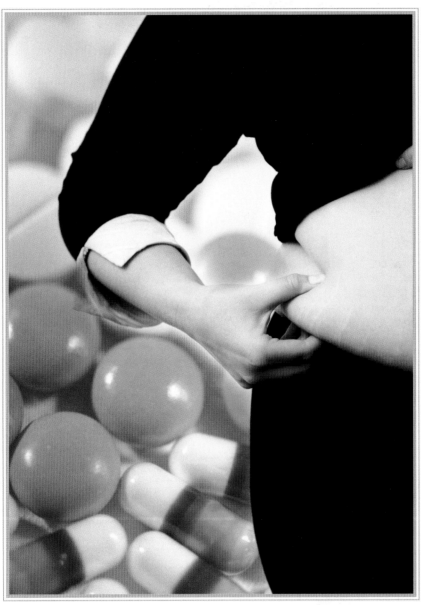

Being overweight is an American epidemic, and many people look to medication as the solution to their problem. Stimulants cause people to burn more calories while they decrease the appetite, both of which help people to lose weight.

How Do Psychostimulants Work?

To understand how these drugs work, you first need some idea of how the brain itself works. The human brain includes, among other things, billions of specialized cells called neu-

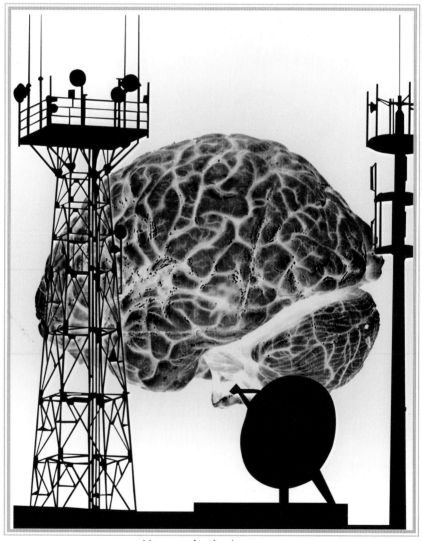

Brain cells are the body's transmitters.

rons. These cells in the brain allow a person to learn, to think, and to remember. Whenever you feel or think anything, millions of neurons are communicating with one another.

Neurotransmitters are what allow this communication to take place. This word's prefix—"neuro-"—refers to nerves and the nervous system, while a "transmitter" is a device that sends information from one place to another. Television and radio stations, for example, have powerful electronic transmitters to broadcast their signals. A television remote control is another, smaller example of a transmitter.

Neurotransmitters are chemicals that send information across the gap, or synapse, between one nerve cell and another, or between a nerve cell and a muscle. The body stores the neurotransmitters in axons, which are found at the end of nerve cells. When an electrical impulse traveling along the nerve reaches the axon, it releases the neurotransmitter, which then moves across the synapse. Some neurotransmitters increase that impulse, while others decrease it. Scientists have identified approximately 300 neurotransmitters in the human body.

Amphetamines increase the body's production of a neurotransmitter called dopamine. This neurotransmitter affects the brain processes that determine emotional responses, movement, and the ability to experience both pleasure and pain. Increased dopamine in the system stimulates both the mind and the body, and it's this mental and physical stimulation that allows people to stay awake, stay focused, and even lose weight. This stimulation also makes people feel better about themselves and thus makes it useful as an antidepressant.

Doctors aren't quite sure exactly how Ritalin works. According to the *Physician's Desk Reference,* "the mode of action in man is not completely understood," but they suspect that it works slightly differently than amphetamines. While amphetamines make the body produce more neurotransmit-

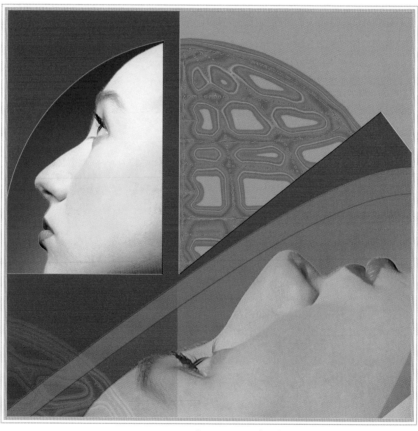

Dopamine influences the brain's pleasure and pain responses.

ters, Ritalin apparently keeps the body from absorbing the neurotransmitters it already has.

These drugs are powerful and effective chemicals—but like any drugs, they bring with them a variety of risks and possible side effects.

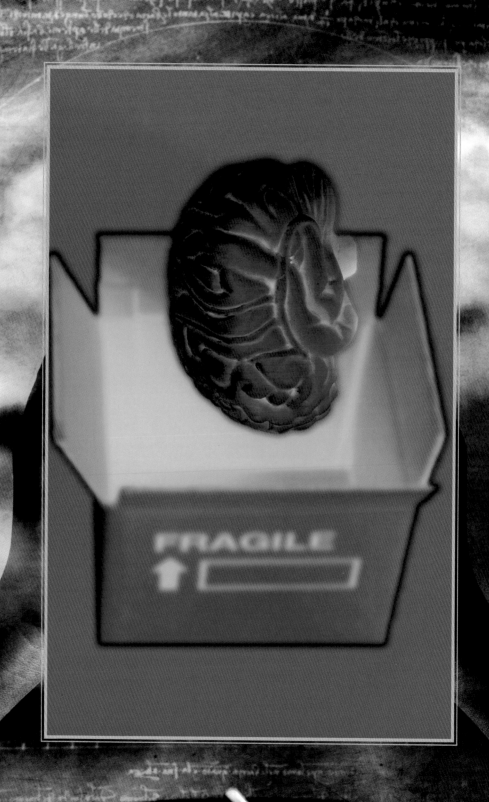

Chapter 4

The Side Effects and Risks of Psychostimulants

lthough psychostimulants have been used effectively as antidepressants in certain situations, doctors have been very hesitant to prescribe them for patients with depression because of their many side effects, and because of the risks involved in taking them for more than a few weeks or months. Doctors also have concerns about these drugs' addictive nature. With the elderly and terminally ill patients, the risks of not taking psychostimulants as antidepressants outweigh these long-term risks. But that's not the case in most depressed patients.

On the other hand, there are other situations in which the benefits of the drugs outweigh the potential risks. Such is the case when treating people diagnosed with ADHD. Most of what we know about the risks of long-term usage of psycho-stimulants comes from looking at the experiences of people with ADHD.

ADHD

ADHD is defined by these main qualities: selective attention, distractibility, impulsivity, and hyperactivity.

Someone with selective attention will go from one extreme to the other; she might have trouble, for instance, concentrating in the classroom when she's bored at school, but she'll

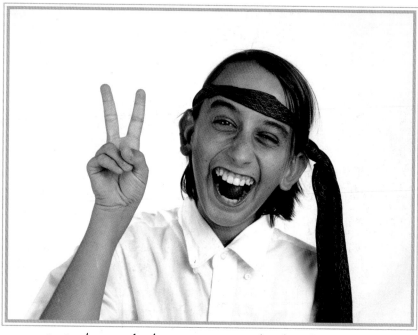

A student who has ADHD may be the class clown as a result of his distractibility, impulsivity, and hyperactivity. Teachers often mislabel such a student a "bad" or poorly behaved youngster.

be able to concentrate for hours at home on something she enjoys.

The second quality of people diagnosed with ADHD is that they are easily distracted: They may start a number of things and never finish any of them. The smallest thing, like a bug crawling up a wall, might command their attention and make them forget what they were doing. Someone with ADHD might be staring out the window at school and get so interested in someone walking down the street that he doesn't hear a thing his teacher says.

People with ADHD are also impulsive. They often act before they consider the consequences of their action or about

sychostimulants and ADHD

the 1930s, teachers at a school for children with "nervous disorders" iticed that the students who were given Benzedrine for their headaches arted doing much better in class than they had been doing. The ildren noticed the difference themselves, and they started to call their nzedrine pills their "arithmetic pills." Charles Bradley, a doctor there, blished an article describing how fourteen of the thirty students owed a "spectacular change in behavior" and "remarkably improved hool performance" after just one week on Benzedrine. According to the nerican Journal of Psychiatry, Bradley's observation "now stands among e most important psychiatric treatment discoveries."

what others might think. As a result, they might have more accidents than other people because they do things like run across the street without looking. This impulsive behavior might also make them more likely to lose things like pens or backpacks because they suddenly put them down without thinking about what they're doing.

A person with ADHD is also hyperactive. In other words, he is fidgety and has trouble sitting still. Teachers may describe him as having a "motor running in high gear inside him." As a result, detailed projects are difficult for him to

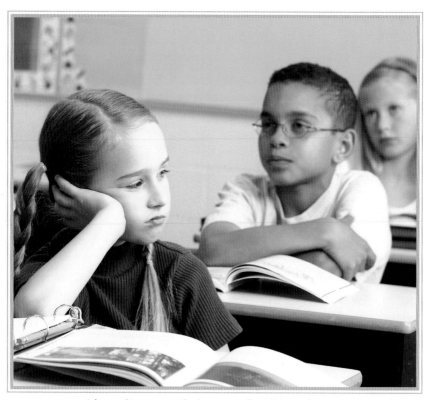

Because of her distractibility, a child with ADHD is often bored in school and has difficulty focusing on the lesson.

complete, and his energy level contributes to his distractibility.

From the perspectives of many doctors, teachers, and parents, controlling this disorder is very important so that a child can do well in school. As a result, children with ADHD are often prescribed a psychostimulant to help them focus their energies on their schoolwork.

The first drug used to treat people with ADHD was Ritalin. Many people find it hard to understand why an amphetamine like Ritalin can help calm someone down. It doesn't seem to make sense. Some think it has this effect because when a person has ADHD, the parts of the brain that affect attention and impulse control are somehow underaroused. The fidgeting and other inappropriate behavior these people display are ways, then, of arousing those parts of the mind. By increasing the body's production of neurotransmitters, amphetamines stimulate those parts of the brain and allow the person to calm down, to concentrate more fully, and to better control their impulsive behavior.

Doctors are very aware of the possible side effects Ritalin might have, and they take care in finding the right dose. Usually, a child starts by taking one 5-milligram pill each day for the first three days, then two pills together for the next three days. Three days at the same dose is usually long enough to notice the drug's effects. Doctors then decide whether to increase the dose or to leave it as it is. If necessary, another pill is added every fourth day until the child reaches a maximum of 20 milligrams per dose. The main purpose of this approach

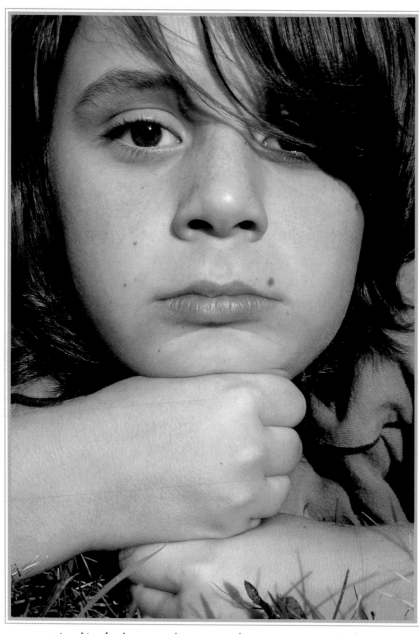

Ritalin helps students with ADHD control their symptoms so that they behave appropriately in a classroom setting; this also enables them to have the opportunity to learn more efficiently.

is to find the best possible response at the lowest possible dose. A second purpose is to minimize any possible side effects.

During these first few weeks, doctors also establish the frequency that a child will take his dosage. The effects of Ritalin last about three to four hours, and many children do quite well in school on one dose early in the morning. Others, however, begin to lose focus in the afternoon, or become hyperactive. For these children, doctors will often prescribe a second dose at noon. This is why, in many schools, students are lined up during the lunch hour to receive their drug from the school nurse. Finding the right frequency is as important as finding the right dosage in balancing the good Ritalin can do with the harm it might do.

Side Effects of Ritalin and Other Psychostimulants

Even with these precautions, however, the risks remain. Ritalin, for example, has several known side effects, even when taken in the right dosage and frequency. Some of these side effects are relatively mild. They include:

1. difficulty sleeping (insomnia)
2. nervousness
3. drowsiness
4. dizziness
5. headaches
6. blurred vision
7. tics (repetitive motions)
8. abdominal pain

9. nausea

10. vomiting

11. decreased appetite

12. weight loss

13. slower weight gain and/or growth

Other side effects, however, are more serious. Some people are allergic to Ritalin and find that after taking it, they have trouble breathing. Sometimes their throats close up, and sometimes their lips or tongue or face swell up. Some come down with hives. Ritalin makes some people's hearts beat irregularly. It makes other people's hearts beat very fast. Some people experience chest pains or very high blood pressure. It can make people feel confused or cause them to act in an unusual way. It can also cause liver damage.

Ritalin and amphetamines such as Dexedrine and Adderall may cause depression, sadness, *lethargy*, and crying among children. In addition, these drugs can induce *obsessions* and *compulsions*, overfocusing, abnormal movements including tics, growth suppression, brain and heart abnormalities, and a variety of other problems.

For instance, when Ryan Raskin was in third grade, he was diagnosed with ADHD and was placed on Ritalin, 20 milligrams every day. In less than a month, his weight dropped from sixty-one pounds to fifty. This weight loss weakened him so much that he was more vulnerable to sicknesses; he contracted *mononucleosis* and his parents had to take him out of school. His doctor reduced his daily dosage to 5 milli-

Dexedrine and the Air Force

Pilots in the U.S. Air Force are sometimes prescribed amphetamines like Dexedrine to help them stay awake during long flights. "It is the gold standard for anti-fatigue," says Colonel Peter Demitry, chief of the U.S. Air Force surgeon-general's science and technology division. "We know that fatigue in aviation kills. . . . This is a life-and-death insurance policy that saves lives." The pilots call Dexedrine their "go-pills," and, according to Colonel Demitry, these drugs have "never been associated with a proven adverse outcome in a military operation. This is a common, legal, ethical, moral and correct application."

grams, and he felt fine when he began fourth grade. That year "was a great year, at school and at home," his mother said.

Fifth grade, though, was different. "It was as if he went through a personality change," his mother said. "He'd come home from school at 4 P.M. and have tantrums that grew increasingly violent. He became dysfunctional at home and in sports. Ryan was devastated and the whole family was frightened because we never knew what to expect day to day, minute to minute." She later discovered that Ryan's mood swings were being caused by his daily withdrawal from the drug. Rather than change his medication, though, or increase his dose, his mother took him completely off Ritalin and began looking for a drug-free alternative. "I was desperate," she said.

DARE

DARE is an acronym for "Drug Abuse Resistance Education." It was begun in 1983 by Los Angeles Police Chief Daryl Gates. In a DARE program, a police officer comes to a public school classroom to teach students the skills they need to avoid involvement in drugs, gangs, and violence. Students usually experience a DARE program in fifth or sixth grade. More than 80 percent of American school districts, and more than fifty-four nations around the world, have DARE programs, and it reaches about thirty-six million students every year.

"If Ritalin had been working, if Ryan were well and happy, I wouldn't be searching for something else."

A story in the *Cincinnati Post*, tells about another child on Ritalin. Tyler Malicoat was diagnosed with ADHD when he was four years old. When he was in preschool, his teacher told his mother, Andrea, that even though Tyler was high strung and active, he was the brightest child in her class. She warned Mrs. Malicoat that other teachers would try to calm him down and recommend that he take Ritalin, but, according to Mrs. Malicoat, "She told me not to listen to them, that Tyler was just fine." Another teacher thought differently, though. She said Tyler was "out of control." From her perspective, he was too imaginative, undisciplined, and unfocused.

And certainly Tyler was causing trouble at home. He was hitting their pet dog as well as striking other members of the family. "You could just see the frustration in him," says his mother. "I was getting so tired of yelling, and I don't think he even understood that what he was doing was wrong."

His parents resisted at first when their family doctor suggested putting Tyler on Ritalin. They didn't want people thinking they'd "drugged up" their child. Eventually, though, they agreed.

The change in Tyler was remarkable, they said. Before, he wouldn't listen and seemed determined to get into trouble.

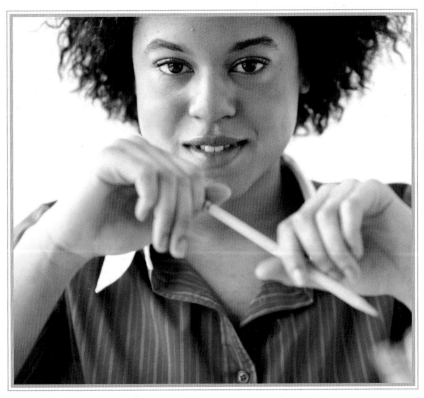

Ritalin is not the answer for every child who happens to be bored with school. ADHD is a diagnosis that should be made with care by professionals.

With Ritalin, he was more agreeable. He was calm and polite and paid attention when he should have. Even Tyler was aware of the difference. He would call the pills he took his "be-good" pills.

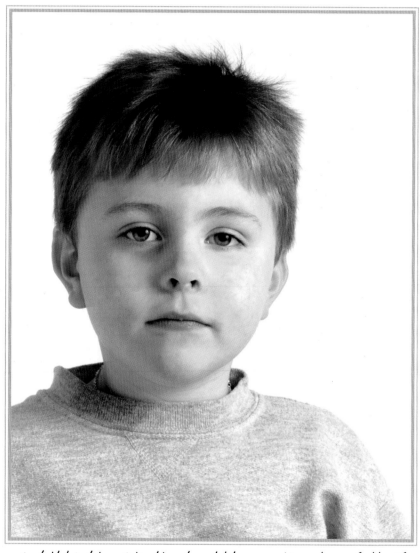

A child taking Ritalin should be monitored carefully. If he seems dull, glassy, and "drugged," there's a problem.

But that doesn't mean he liked them. In fact, he hated almost everything about them. He hated the way they tasted and the way they made him feel. He even hated that everyone was always asking him if he'd taken his medicine.

"It's hard to know what to do, what's right for him," said Mrs. Malicoat. "My mother won't watch him if he hasn't taken his Ritalin. And when I tried to take him off, his teachers complained."

When Tyler was on Ritalin, he was calm and quiet, smiling and responding politely to questions. But the way he answered, and the way he moved, was very slow, dull, and deliberate. His eyes were glassy and unfocused, and he seemed to do everything in slow motion.

His mother hated seeing him like this. "Whenever he takes his medicine," she said, "he just looks stoned. I have him on the lowest dosage, and still, he's just out of it."

Like Ryan, Tyler was smaller than he should have been. Tyler often didn't want to eat because the pills "make my belly hurt." In addition, he became scared of shadows and empty rooms. He wouldn't go upstairs or down into the basement by himself anymore.

"Some days, I think Tyler wouldn't need the medication if he had constant attention," said Mrs. Malicoat. "But who has the time?"

Although it can be difficult to live with these kinds of side effects, many people do without experiencing any further problems. Sometimes, though, something more serious may be taking place. Take Stephanie Hall, for instance, whose story was told on *Hard Copy* and the Web site www.kats-korner.com/health/ritalin.html. She began taking Ritalin when she was in first grade. The medication did seem to help her do well in school, but she experienced various side effects—stomachaches, nausea, and especially headaches, which she had every day. These symptoms only stopped on the weekends, when she didn't take any Ritalin. As she went through second and third grade, her doctors would vary her dosage. They wanted to find a balance between getting the good result they wanted while avoiding her daily headaches, but the headaches continued.

When she was in fourth grade, however, she started doing strange things now and then. One day, for instance, she ran away from the child-care center where she went after school. Her mother, Janet, said, "They chased her but couldn't catch her. She yelled 'I'm 10 and a half now.' She took off across a busy five-lane road, bought her grandmother a paper, and took it all the way downtown where she worked. Day-care workers were screaming at her to come to them. Her DARE officer couldn't believe she acted like [that]. They called me at work. I never worked after school hours again."

That summer Stephanie didn't take any Ritalin at all. Her mother remembers that in August:

suddenly she zoned out on me . . . totally disconnected. She said, "Mom I love you." We always told each other this, so I thought nothing of it. But then she said it again and she had this empty stare on her face. I said, "Steph, what's the matter?" and she said, "I see her again." I said, who? She said,

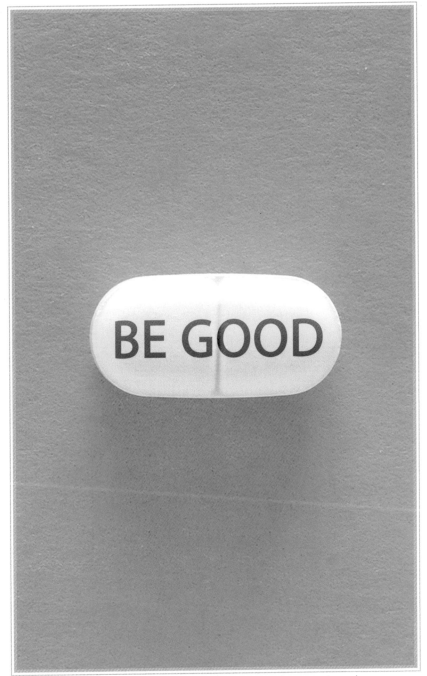

Ritalin should not be viewed as a simple
solution to behavior problems.

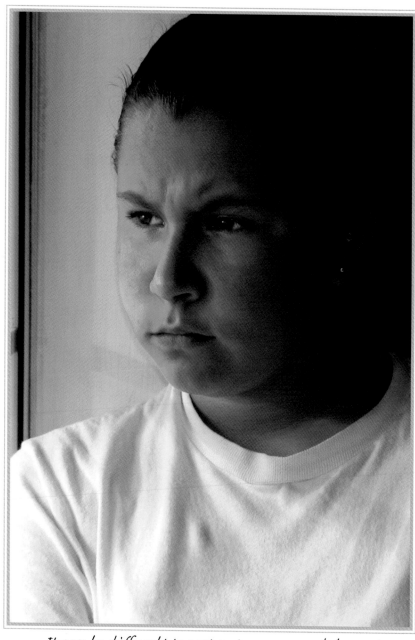

It can be difficult to sort out common adolescent issues from more dangerous warning symptoms. Sometimes, parents would prefer to blame a medication for their teens' problems than to look deeper.

"The angel . . . she looks mad." Then she snapped out of it. She said the angel had white and red all around her. Some of the angels were blue. And they all had four wings. It reminds me of when she was first put on Ritalin back in the first and second grade and told me of seeing angels then.

When school started again in the fall, Stephanie went back on Ritalin. Things seemed fine until the day in October when the school's vice principal called. Stephanie had been swearing—something her mother says was "totally out of character" for her. Apparently, another girl had tried to take her lunch money. A few days later, Janet Hall heard her daughter swearing again, this time at a boy after school. "I was shocked," she said. "I grounded her. Then, her grades started going down . . . mostly D's."

By December, Stephanie had F's. Her mother talked to their pediatrician, and despite the daily migraine headaches that she continued to have every day, they decided to double Stephanie's daily dosage when school started up again in January. She seemed "spaced out" the morning she took her first increased dose, her mother said, but when she came home she seemed fine.

The very next morning, though, Stephanie was dead. She had died in her sleep. The coroner said she had died of "natural causes" six days before her twelfth birthday.

Stephanie had a variety of health issues; the fact that she was taking Ritalin may have been only a coincidence. However, stories like this have led to the creation of outspoken parents' groups that blame Ritalin for a host of dangerous side effects. They claim that Stephanie is not the only child to have died apparently from taking Ritalin over a long period of time.

For instance, Matthew Smith was six years old and in the first grade when he was diagnosed with ADHD. (You can read more about Matthew at www.cbsnews.com/stories/2000/04/18/national/main185425.shtml.) His parents say they were told that Ritalin "was a very mild medication and would stimulate the brain stem and help Matthew focus."

"He said 'I don't want to take it, it makes me feel stoned,'" his father said. "He took it because we told him he needed to take it." But on March 21, 2000, Matthew died suddenly of a heart attack. He had taken Ritalin every day for eight years—more than half his life. His death certificate listed the cause of his death as "long term use of methylphenidate (Ritalin)." An autopsy showed that his heart had "clear signs of small vessel damage" caused by his long-term use of the drug. It also showed that it had caused his heart to grow larger by age fourteen than that of a full-grown man.

There may be other dangers associated with long-term Ritalin use. In 2005, the federal government announced it had begun to investigate a claim by a small Texas study that indicated children who use Ritalin may face an increased risk of cancer later in life. The study found damage to the *chromosomes* of twelve children who had taken Ritalin for three months. Drugs already known to cause cancer cause similar types of damage.

Other Psychostimulants

Adderall is another psychostimulant that is often prescribed for people diagnosed with ADHD. The FDA approved it for use in 1996. While it has some of the same potential side effects as Ritalin, such as closing of the throat and abnormal

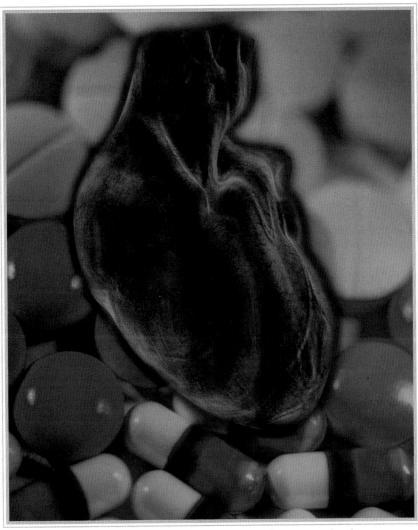

Prolonged use of stimulants can damage the heart.

behavior, it can also cause hallucinations. Some of its minor side effects are insomnia and diarrhea.

In February 2005, the Canadian government pulled Adderall from the market after it was linked to the sudden deaths of twelve American boys. All twelve died between 1999 and 2003. The youngest was seven years old and the oldest was sixteen. They had taken Adderall for as little as one day to as long as eight years.

Although the American FDA had the same information as Health Canada, they did not remove the drug from the market. According to Russell Katz, director of the FDA's **neuro-**

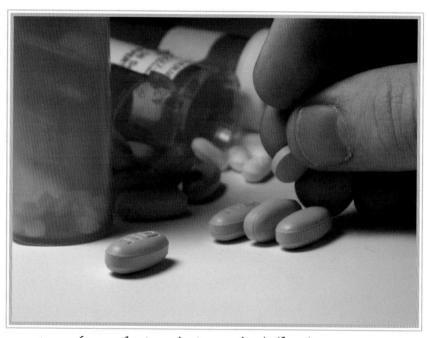

Even for professionals, it can be difficult to sort out all the factors that contribute to a tragedy. Because a person who dies is taking a medication does not necessarily mean that the medicine caused his death.

logical drugs office, because five of the children who died had known heart defects, Adderall may not have been the reason they died. In addition, many of the other seven children had "unusual circumstances" that made the link to Adderall hard to establish. "One child was in a boot camp and exercising in 110 degrees," he said.

> Two others had high blood levels of the drug, possibly reflecting an overdose. The way we try to assess causality—to ask, "Did the drug do this?"—it is hard to answer that by looking at an individual case. Just because a child died while on Adderall doesn't mean the drug was the cause. It could have been fifty different causes.

In August of 2005, Health Canada allowed Adderall back on the market, saying that a panel of experts had decided that they didn't have enough evidence that Adderall had caused the deaths.

Another psychostimulant, Cylert, was withdrawn from the U.S. market in March of 2005. The consumer group Public Citizen reported that thirteen people had died since 1975 from liver problems traced to taking the drug. Another 193 patients had suffered "serious consequences." An analysis done by the FDA showed that Cylert increased the risk of liver failure by almost seventeen times.

Research also indicates that stimulants do cause a slightly increased risk of sudden death from cardiac issues. What's more, stimulants can bring on the onset of psychosis in some cases. If a person with a bipolar mood disorder was to take

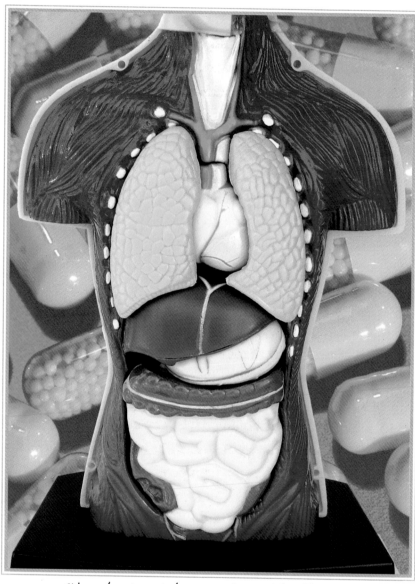

Stimulants can have serious side effects on various important body functions.

a stimulant, her condition could easily be kicked up a notch into a manic episode. These are all risk factors that must be considered when doctors prescribe psychostimulants.

Psychostimulants and Depression

Care must always be taken when blaming a drug for particular "side effects." In some cases, the deaths and other serious consequences may be more related to the initial condition that caused the drug to be prescribed; in other cases, sheer coincidence can build a negative image in the public's opinion, one that is not necessarily built on a sound ***statistical*** foundation.

Still, it's no wonder that doctors shy away from prescribing psychostimulants as antidepressants except under certain circumstances. Although these drugs can be effective in helping to ease the symptoms of depression, the possible risks of taking such a drug over a number of years often outweigh any possible benefits. Another major problem with psychostimulants is that they have a high potential for abuse.

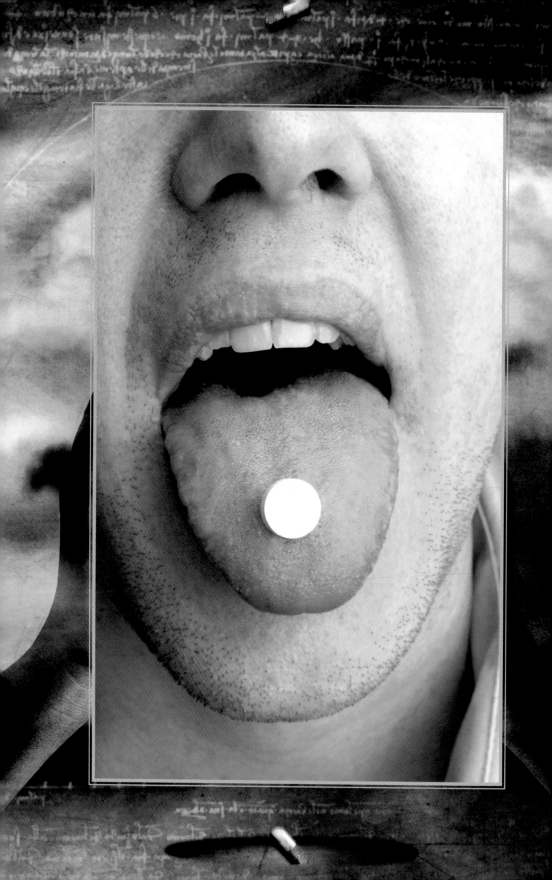

Chapter 5

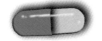

Psychostimulant Abuse

he U.S. government lists psychostimulants as "Schedule II" drugs, which means there's a good chance these drugs may be abused. The Drug Enforcement Agency (DEA) classifies all federally regulated drugs according to five schedules. Schedule I includes drugs that, in its opinion, have both a high potential for abuse and no accepted medical use. Such drugs as heroin, marijuana, and lysergic acid diethylamide (LSD) appear on Schedule I. Schedule II includes drugs that also have a high potential for abuse but also have an accepted medical use. Among Schedule II drugs are morphine, cocaine, and methamphetamine. Ritalin and Adderall are also on that list, and have become two of the most commonly abused drugs in America.

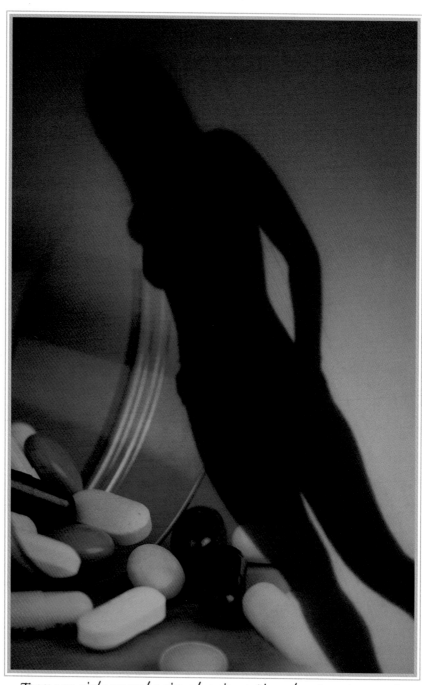

Teenage girls may begin abusing stimulants as a way to conform to our culture's standard for female beauty.

The Center on Addiction and Substance Abuse at Columbia University reported in July 2005, "Our nation is in the throes of an epidemic of controlled prescription drug abuse and addiction." It went on to say that, "From 1992 to 2003, abuse of controlled prescription drugs grew at a rate twice that of marijuana abuse; five times that of cocaine abuse; sixty times that of heroin abuse." About 14 percent of high school seniors have used prescription drugs for nonmedical reasons, with about 10 percent abusing either Ritalin or Adderall. A January 2005 survey of over 2,000 students from 119 four-year colleges in the United States showed that the use of psychostimulants like Ritalin and Adderall for nonmedical use had increased by 3 percent over 2004.

Some of this abuse stems from girls' desire to lose weight and conform to society's concept of "pretty." Take Lauren, for example, who tells her story in the October 2005 issue of *Girls' Life*. All through middle school, Lauren was unhappy with her body. "Every time I was in the hallways," she says, "there was always a girl who was skinnier or prettier. I wanted to be the 'hottest' girl. I felt if all the guys were looking at me, it would boost my self-esteem." So, when she was fourteen, she started taking drugs, hoping they would help make her thin and help her fit in at school.

"The first drug I tried was pot," she says, "but, about two months later, I started taking Adderall, Concerta, and Ritalin, which are all drugs for ADHD. Everyone I knew seemed to have them—either by prescription, or their parents or siblings had them—so they gave them to me. I knew those drugs would decrease my appetite."

Hazelden Foundation

The Hazelden Foundation began in a farmhouse by a lake in Minnesota back in 1949. Since then, it has grown into one of the largest alcohol and drug rehabilitation centers in the world. It has served millions of people from every state in the Union and from forty-two foreign countries. Hazelden was one of the first organizations to offer a multidisciplinary approach to overcoming addiction. On average, more than half of Hazelden's graduates stay off drugs and alcohol for more than a year after they finish, with another 35 percent significantly reducing their use. Between 70 and 80 percent report that they have improved the quality of their lives and that they have seen positive changes in their relationships with others, in their job performance, and in their ability to handle problems.

By the time Lauren was sixteen, though, the drugs began causing her a great deal of trouble. "My life felt totally out of control," she says.

I was so depressed, and sick and tired of my life being all about drugs. I was always lying to my parents, trying to keep track of the lies and hiding everything from them. It was exhausting. I had been a straight-A student but, by that point, I had fallen to a 2.4 GPA. I stopped caring about anything but drugs. One day, I cut my wrists to end it all. My parents found me and rushed me to the hospital. They had no idea I was addicted to drugs until that day. Soon after, I was sent to rehab. It changed my life. It taught me self-acceptance.

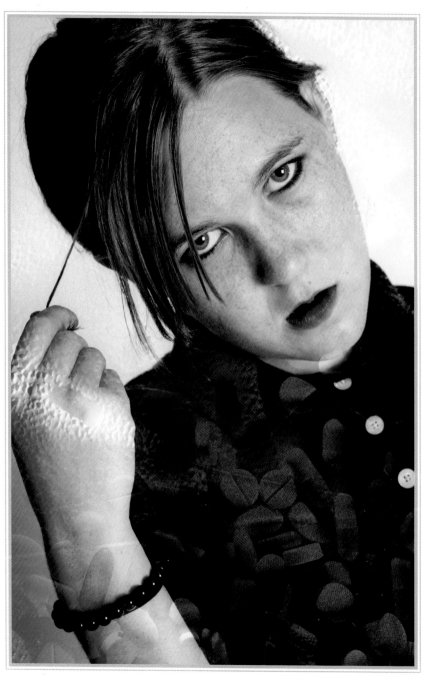

When teens self-medicate, their drug abuse ultimately only adds further serious complications to their lives.

Part of the reason people abuse psychostimulants is because they are so easily available. According to Carol Falkowski, director of research communications at the Hazelden Foundation in Minnesota, "We live in a world where five million

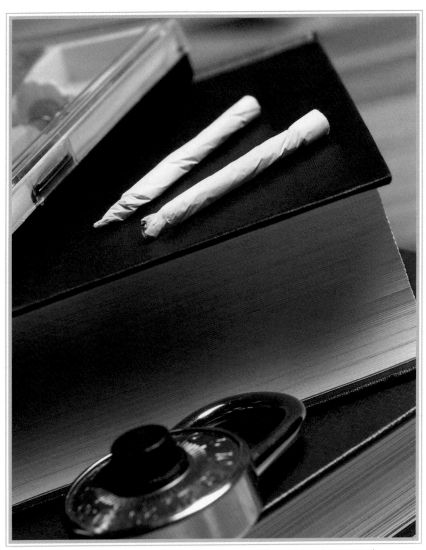

Marijuana is still a popular adolescent drug—but Ritalin is becoming more and more popular as well.

school-age children take a prescription drug for behavior disorders, so kids learn at an early age that pills change moods. There are pills all around as they grow up, so they do not see them as anything inherently dangerous." Girls in particular find the drugs tempting because stimulants can help them lose weight. Falkowski says girls "are so concerned with body image by middle school. There's just so much pressure around them to be thin."

Some people, particularly young adults, use psychostimulants as they would alcohol or marijuana. A DEA study done in 2000 of drug treatment centers in Wisconsin, Indiana, and South Carolina found that 30 to 50 percent of the people there said they had used Ritalin to get high. Jacob Stone, a student at Sobriety High School, a drug treatment school in Minneapolis, says, "I'd take six, seven, eight pills at a time. I'd snort them. Along the way, I knew a couple who would melt them down and shoot them up." He started misusing Ritalin after he was diagnosed with ADHD while in sixth grade. Eventually, he began selling his pills to others. "The people who were most interested in it were the younger kids who weren't trying to do real drugs," he said. "They wanted something that seemed like it was okay to do and that still would give them a good buzz." Another Sobriety High student, Abby Neff, said, "I know people that stay up for days off Adderall or Ritalin, and it does the same thing as coke."

Unfortunately, parents often have no idea what their children are doing. "My mom never had an inkling that I was using Ritalin to get high," says Jacob and Abby's classmate,

Wyeth Gibson. They're also often unaware of the drug's potential for abuse. Lynda S. Madison of the Creighton University Medical School in Omaha, Nebraska, says, "I have known parents who said they took the Ritalin prescribed for their child themselves, or gave it to their other children, 'just to see if it helps.' Unfortunately, as useful as the medication is for children who truly have ADHD, it often is seen as completely **benign** and readily accessible."

In May of 2000, the DEA's "Drugs of Concern" bulletin listed Ritalin alongside cocaine, LSD, and ecstasy. Deputy Director Terrance Woodworth testified before Congress that "continued increases in the medical prescription of these drugs without the appropriate safeguards . . . can only lead to increased stimulant abuse among U.S. children." Another indication of increasing stimulant abuse is the rise in the number of drug-related emergency room visits. In 1999, there were 261 amphetamine-related emergency room visits. By 2003, that number had increased to 1,355.

Some who abuse psychostimulants use them to help them focus on their schoolwork and study longer and more effectively. A senior at Los Altos High School in California says that taking Adderall is "like caffeine or Red Bull." He says that it helps him focus on his finals and on his major papers, adding, "It's like any other pick-me-up."

Another senior, this one at Palo Alto High School, says that he continues to take Adderall even though "I know it's probably messing up my body." The pills have given him sleepless nights, chills, and a racing heart. He's even lost weight because of them. But he says they help him manage the demands of his schoolwork, sports, and his busy social life.

Rachel Berman, who wrote about Adderall for the Los Altos High School newspaper, says that "It's happening more and more and it helps people understand how much pressure is put on kids my age to succeed."

And the pressure that begins in high school continues in college. In the United States, an average of 7 percent of college students misuse drugs like Ritalin and Adderall to help them study. At some colleges, the percentage is as high as 25 percent. Generally, these rates were higher in the Northeast, where the Ivy League schools are located, and at colleges "with more competitive admission standards." And according to Dr. Henry Wechsler of the Harvard School of Public Health, "while much is known about the college study use of

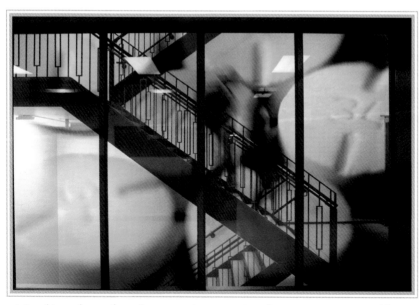

Ritalin abuse has become increasingly common in colleges.

alcohol, cigarettes, marijuana and other illicit drugs, we've not had a handle on the abuse of prescription drugs."

Jenna is an undergraduate at Yale, one of the most competitive universities in the United States. She says, "Adderall is the drug that works the best. It helps you concentrate more than either Dex [Dexedrine] or Ritalin, and you feel physically better on it than any other ADHD medication." Although she has no prescription and has not been diagnosed with ADHD, Jenna takes ten to twenty milligrams of Adderall every day. Sometimes at night, she takes even more—sixty to ninety milligrams, well above the recommended amount. She says she needs it to work effectively. "I can do work without it," she says, "but my concentration is just not there."

Ivy League

The Ivy League is a group of eight universities, all located in the Northeast: Harvard, Yale, Princeton, Dartmouth, Brown, Cornell, Columbia, and Penn. All but Cornell were founded before the American Revolution. All of them are privately run universities, although Cornell has several state-supported colleges. These are some of the most competitive schools in the United States. For example, only about 17 percent of those who apply to Yale are accepted for admission. In 2006, tuition at these universities averaged about $45,000 a year.

During finals in 2004, Jenna went on an Adderall binge. "There was a time when I saw the sunrise every day," she says. "By the end of that, your heart starts feeling weak. After three days of no sleep, I started hallucinating. You get anxiety attacks."

She knows Adderall isn't good for her. She has pain in her sinuses and has considered the possibility of lesions on her brain. She and her friends have tried to cut back. Generally, students at Yale think of Adderall as a "less-severe, less-intense drug." But she now wishes she had never gotten started on it. "If I would go back to when we first tried it," she says, "I might not have bought it. It's like any drug; it does become addictive."

Clearly, psychostimulants carry with them a risk that they may be abused. When it comes to the use of psychostimulant medications to treat depression, this risk must be considered. It's one more reason why doctors generally only use these medications only as a last resort when it comes to treating depression.

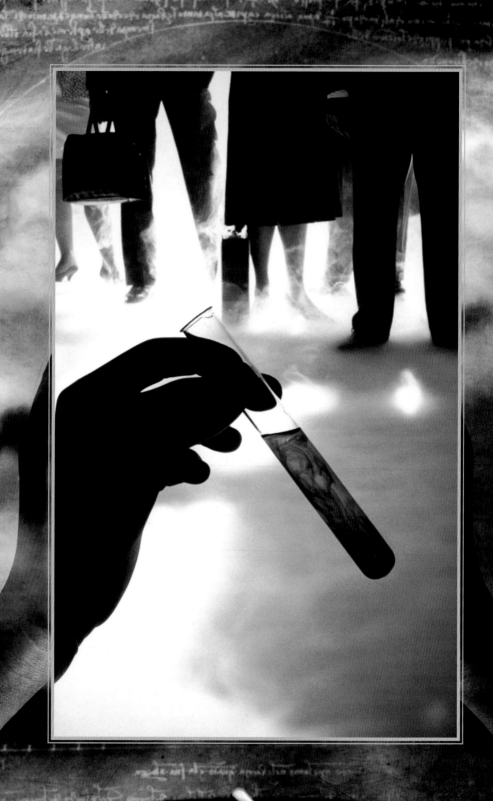

Chapter 6

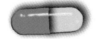

Research and Trends for the Future

Ritalin was created in a search for an amphetamine without the risks and side effects. In many ways, that search failed. Modafinil (Provigil) was created in a search for a Ritalin without the risks and side effects. That search, however, may have succeeded. If there is a future for psychostimulants as antidepressants, it lies with Provigil.

Like other psychostimulants, Provigil boosts alertness, memory, and energy. But because it apparently affects the hypothalamus rather than the central nervous system, it lacks many of the side effects of drugs like Ritalin and Adderall. Users generally do not experience the agitation, irritability, or nervousness other psychostimulants cause. And because it does not cause the *euphoria* that amphetamines can cause, the possibility of addiction is much less. Unlike Ritalin and Adderall, modafinil is listed by the Drug Enforcement Agency as a Schedule IV drug. These drugs have an accepted medical use and a low potential for abuse.

Coping with Depression's Fatigue

One possible use of modafinil in treating depression concerns the fatigue, or weariness, that depression often causes. This can affect individuals' work performance and productivity; it can also make it very difficult for people to take any constructive steps to combat their depression. Unfortunately, the symptoms of fatigue respond slowly to both antidepressants and psychotherapy. As a result, several studies have been conducted to discover if modafinil can relieve this weariness.

Between 2001 and 2003, doctors at Upstate Medical Center in Syracuse, New York, studied twenty men and women with clinical depression. Besides their standard antidepressants, they were also given modafinil. The study found that the combination of modafinil with a standard antidepressant "significantly improved" not only their fatigue but also their depression. They became less sleepy and more energetic. The doctors concluded that this combination of drugs "improved mood and quality of life" in the sixteen patients who finished the study. Other studies, however, indicate that this improvement is only short term.

Post-Stroke Depression

Modafinil may also be useful in treating post-stroke depression. Between 10 and 25 percent of people who suffer a stroke

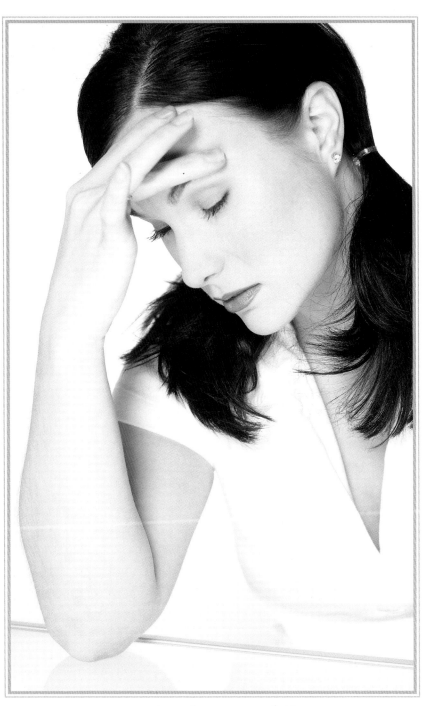

Depression often causes fatigue.

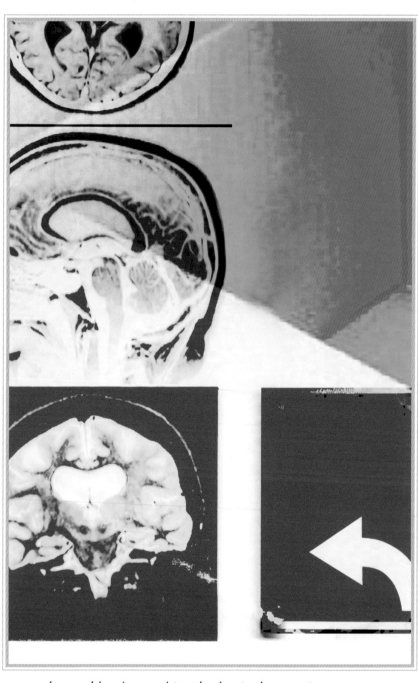

When a blood vessel in the brain bursts, it can cause serious damage to a variety of body functions.

are diagnosed afterward with major depression, with 10 to 40 percent suffering from minor depression. This depression interferes with rehabilitation, increases the possibility of contracting another illness, and makes it more likely that the patient may die. It also increases the possibility of suicide.

In 2004, doctors at the University of California reported on the case of an elderly woman they called "Ms. A." After she regained consciousness following her treatment for stroke, she was disoriented and unable to follow directions. She was also described as not caring what happened anymore and having very little energy. She was alert but spoke very little. The doctors decided to discontinue the antidepressant she had been taking and started giving her 100 milligrams of modafinil every day instead. After her third dose, she became more alert and spontaneously engaged in conversation with

Stroke

A stroke occurs when a blood vessel in the brain either bursts or is blocked by a clot. When that happens, the part of the brain that the vessel services can no longer receive the oxygen it needs and shuts down. Some of the symptoms of stroke are loss of muscle control, slurred speech, and dizziness. Stroke is the third leading cause of death in the United States, after heart attack and cancer. In 2002, more than 160,000 Americans died of stroke.

her doctors. She was able to deal more easily with her physical therapy and as a result was released from the hospital a week earlier than expected.

Bipolar Disorder

Modafinil may also prove useful in treating certain patients suffering from the type of mood disorder known as bipolar disorder. This is sometimes treated with a drug called divalproex. Unfortunately, this drug can leave patients sedated, which may make them avoid taking it.

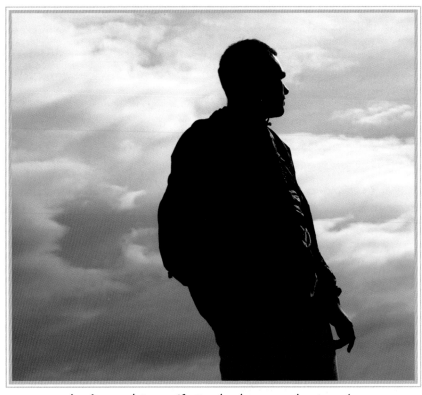

Lack of sunshine affects the human brain; gloomy days can literally make a person depressed.

"John Smith," for instance, was taking 750 milligrams of divalproex every day along with his antidepressant. However, the drug caused him to sleep twelve to fourteen hours a day and made it impossible for him to go to work. His doctors reduced his divalproex dosage to 500 milligrams and suggested he take 100 milligrams of modafinil every day as well. After a week, they increased his modafinil to 200 milligrams a day. His sleeping decreased to eight hours a day, and he didn't feel drowsy during the day. After nine months of unemployment, he became able to find work, and he was also able to participate again in the life of his family. A year later, he was still sleeping normally and had experienced no side effects.

Seasonal Affective Disorder

In France, modafinil has been used successfully to treat seasonal affective disorder (SAD, also known as winter depression). There, forty-six-year-old "Jacques Ste. Pierre" entered a "mood disorder" clinic. For more than twenty years, he had become depressed during the winter only to experience a full recovery in the spring and summer. When the combination of an antidepressant and light therapy failed to help him, his doctors halted the light therapy and in its place started to give him 200 milligrams of modafinil every day. After two weeks, the depression had lifted but he felt very fatigued, so the doctors increased his daily dosage to 300 milligrams. After five weeks, he no longer felt any depression, and he did not experience any fatigue. Because this improvement took place after ten weeks on an antidepressant, and since he improved two full months before the coming of spring, his doctors declared that "this improvement may be primarily or even exclusively attributed to modafinil."

ADHD

Finally, modafinil may soon be accepted as a treatment for ADHD. A study in 2005 involving almost 250 patients with ADHD showed that it improved their symptoms. "Children and adolescents treated with once-daily (modafinil) showed improvement in ADHD symptoms, including inattention, impulsivity, and hyperactivity, both at school and at home," said researcher Joseph Biederman of Boston's Massachusetts

Seasonal Affective Disorder

Many people find the short, dark, cold days of late fall and winter to be somewhat depressing. But when people experience very strong and powerful sadness as a result of this, psychiatrists say that they suffer from seasonal affective disorder (SAD), also known as winter depression. People with SAD lack energy, crave sleep, and develop a craving for sweets, often resulting in weight gain. It's believed that as many as ten million Americans experience SAD every year. Seventy to 80 percent of those affected are women. Since it's thought that lack of light causes the disorder, one type of treatment for SAD is light therapy, using a box that exposes the individual to bright light for thirty minutes or more each day.

General Hospital. Also, there were few side effects reported, although 29 percent of the patients said they had trouble sleeping, and 16 percent said that the drug decreased their appetite.

There have not yet been studies comparing the effects of modafinil with Ritalin and Adderall. According to James T. Perrin, an expert in the treatment of ADHD, "We don't yet know if modafinil is any better or worse than these medications. What we do know is that this medication does seem to work in children with ADHD in the usual ways." The use of modafinil to treat the millions with ADHD, however, may prove much safer than the use of Ritalin and Adderall. It may also help reduce the amount of abuse of those drugs.

It's possible, of course, that eventually researchers may learn that modafinil, like Dexedrine and Ritalin before it, also has risks and side effects. It is, after all, a relatively new drug, and it sometimes takes many years before the true risks of a drug are fully known.

Further Reading

Ainsworth, Patricia. *Understanding Depression.* Jackson: University Press of Mississippi, 2000.

Machoian, Lisa. *The Disappearing Girl: Learning the Language of Teenage Depression.* New York: Dutton, 2005.

Merrell Kenneth W. *Helping Students Overcome Depression and Anxiety: A Practical Guide.* New York: Guilford, 2001.

Mondimore, Francis Mark. *Adolescent Depression: A Guide for Parents.* Baltimore, Md.: Johns Hopkins, 2002.

Shenk, Joshua Wolf. *Lincoln's Melancholy: How Depression Challenged a President and Fueled His Greatness.* Boston: Houghton Mifflin, 2005.

Turkington, Carol, and Eliot F. Kaplan. *Making the Antidepressant Decision: How to Choose the Right Treatment Option for You or Your Loved One.* Chicago: Contemporary Books, 2001.

Zucker, Faye. *Depression.* New York: Watts, 2003.

For More Information

Amphetamines
www.amphetamines.com

Depression Information and Treatment
www.psychologyinfo.com/depression

Drug Enforcement Administration
www.dea.gov

Drug Information Online
www.drugs.com

Drugs and the Brain: Stimulants
www.csusm.edu/DandB/stimulants.html

National Institute of Mental Health
www.nimh.nih.gov

National Institute on Drug Abuse
www.nida.nih.gov

Provigil (modafinil)
www.provigil.com

Publisher's note:
The Web sites listed on this page were active at the time of publication. The publisher is not responsible for Web sites that have changed their addresses or discontinued operation since the date of publication. The publisher will review and update the Web-site list upon each reprint.

Glossary

anhedonia: The inability to experience pleasure.

apathy: Lack of interest in anything.

benign: Of no danger to health.

chromosomes: Body material that contains hereditary information.

compulsions: Irrational forces that make someone do something.

congestive heart failure: A form of heart failure characterized by the heart's inability to pump away blood fast enough to avoid the veins becoming over-filled.

delusional: Believing things that are not true.

diffident: Lacking self-confidence, shy.

electroconvulsive therapy: The passing of a small electrical current through the brain to cause a seizure, used in treating severe psychiatric disorders such as depression.

euphoria: A feeling of great joy, excitement, or well-being.

hallucinate: Seeing, hearing, or otherwise sensing things that are not really there.

ideation: The process of forming and relating ideas.

lesions: Wounds or injuries.

lethargy: A state of physical slowness and mental dullness caused by fatigue, disease, or drugs.

melancholy: Affected with or marked by depression of the spirit; sad.

mononucleosis: An infectious disease characterized by fever and swollen lymph nodes.

neurological: Having to do with the nervous system.

obsessions: The objects of someone's persistent ideas or emotions.

placebo: A substance that looks like a pill or other medicine but contains no medication.

provocative: Deliberately done to excite or annoy people.

psychomotor agitation: Unusually active body movement triggered by mental activity.

psychotherapy: The treatment of mental disorders by psychological methods that include counseling.

schizophrenia: A psychiatric disorder characterized by a loss of contact with reality.

statistical: Having to do with the interpretation of numerical data in terms of samples and populations.

synthetic: Not of natural origin.

Bibliography

"Air Force rushes to defend amphetamine use." *The Age* (January 18, 2003). http://www.theage.com.au/articles/ 2003/01/17/1042520778665.html?oneclick=true.

American Psychological Association. "New Report on Women and Depression." http://www.apa.org/releases/ depressionreport.html.

Baughman, Fred A. "Who Killed Stephanie Hall?" http:// www.kats-korner.com/health/ritalin.html.

Berigan, Tim. "Modafinil Treatment of Excessive Sedation Associated With Divalproex Sodium." *Canadian Journal of Psychiatry* (January 2004). http://www.cpa-apc.org/ Publications/Archives/CJP/2004/January/lettersModafinil. asp.

Block, Susan. "Assessing and Managing Depression in the Terminally Ill Patient." American College of Physicians, February 2000. http://www.acponline.org/ethics/block.htm.

Boyles, Salynn. "Narcolepsy Drug Shows Promise for ADHD." WebMD, December 6, 2005. http://www.webmd. com/content/Article/116/112029.htm.

Bransfield, Robert C. "Potential Uses of Modafinil in Psychiatric Disorders." *The Journal of Applied Research* 4, no. 2 (2004) http://www.jrnlappliedresearch.com/articles/ Vol4Iss2/Bransfield-Jar-spring.pdf.

Breggin, Peter R. *Reclaiming Our Children: A Healing Solution for a Nation in Crisis*. Cambridge: Perseus Books, 2000.

"Caffeine Nation." *CBS News*. http://www.cbsnews.com/stories/2002/11/14/sunday/main529388.shtml.

Centers for Disease Control and Prevention. http://www.cdc.gov/mmwr/preview/mmwrhtml/mm5444a2.htm.

Conte, Andrew. "More Students Abusing Hyperactivity Drugs." *Pittsburgh Tribune-Review*, October 25, 2004. http://pittsburghlive.com/x/tribune-review/trib/regional/s_265518.html.

"Coca Cola History." Solar Navigator. http://www.solarnavigator.net/sponsorship/coca_cola.htm.

DeGrandpre, Richard J. *Ritalin Nation: Rapid-Fire Culture and the Transformation of Human Consciousness*. New York: Norton, 1999.

Diller, Lawrence H. *Running on Ritalin: A Physician Reflects on Children, Society, and Performance in a Pill*. New York: Bantam, 1998.

Drug Enforcement Administration. http://www.dea.gov/pubs/abuse/1-csa.htm#Schedule%20I.

Even, C., S. Friedman, R. Dardennes, and J. D. Guelfi. "Modafinil as an Alternative to Light Therapy for Winter Depression." *European Psychiatry* (2004). http://www.anakata.hack.se/index/referenser/modafinil/eur.psychiatry.19.65-66.2004.pdf.

Feinstein, Jessica. "Adderall: The Academic Steroid." *Yale Daily News Magazine*, January 24, 2005. http://www.yaledailynews.com/article.asp?AID=27960.

Frierson, Robert L., John J. Wey, and James Boswell Tabler. "Psychostimulants for Depression in the Medically Ill." American Family Physician (January 1991). http://www.findarticles.com/p/articles/mi_m3225/is_n1_v43/ai_10365377.

Goodwin, Doris Kearns. *Team of Rivals.* New York: Simon and Schuster, 2005.

Health Canada. http://www.hc-sc.gc.ca/ahc-asc/media/nr-cp/2005/2005_92_e.html.

Healy, David. *The Antidepressant Era.* Cambridge: Harvard University Press, 1997.

Hecht, Joanna. "Campus Prescription Drug Abuse to be Documented." *Trinity Tripod*, October 25, 2005. http://www.trinitytripod.com/media/paper520/news/2005/10/25/News/Campus.Prescription.Drug.Abuse.To.Be.Documented-1033159.shtml.

Horwitz, Allan V., and Jerome C. Wakefield. "The Age of Depression." *Public Interest* (Winter 2005). http://www.findarticles.com/p/articles/mi_m0377/is_158/ai_n8680970.

Leuchter, Andrew. "Clinical Consult in Depression," February 2004. http://www.mhsource.com/depconsult/feb2004.jhtml?_requestid=318012.

Marks, Alexandra. "Schoolyard Hustlers' New Drug: Ritalin." *Christian Science Monitor*, October 31, 2000. http://

csmonitor.com/cgi-bin/durableRedirect.pl?/durable/
2000/10/31/fp1s4-csm.shtml.

National Institute of Mental Health. http://www.nimh.nih.
gov/publicat/nimhdepression.pdf.

National Library of Medicine. http://www.nlm.nih.gov/
medlineplus/druginfo/medmaster/a682188.html.

Nevins, Conor. "Non-Prescription Adderall Use: A Growing
Trend Among College Students." Northeastern University
School of Journalism, December 2004. http://www.
journalism.neu.edu/studentwork/nevins.html.

Patel, Julie. "Before College, High School Students Turn to
Stimulant to Succeed." *Billings Gazette*, June 1, 2005. http://
www.billingsgazette.com/index.php?id = 1&display = redne
ws/2005/06/01/build/health/50-stimulant.inc.

Physicians' Desk Reference. Montvale, N.J.: Thomson, 2005.

Popyk, Lisa. "Ritalin Decision Agonizing." *Cincinnati Post*,
April 15, 2000. http://www.cincypost.com/news/2000/
drugsd041500.html.

"Questions Raised Over Ritalin." *CBS News*. http://www.
cbsnews.com/stories/2000/04/18/national/main185425.
shtml.

Ryan, Sandy. "Prescription for Trouble." *Girls' Life*. October–November 2005.

Schwartz, T. L., N. Azhar, K. Cole, G. Hopkins, N. Nihalani,
M. Simionescu, J. Husain, and N. Jones. "An Open-Label
Study of Adjunctive Modafinil in Patients with Sedation

Related to Serotonergic Antidepressant Therapy." *Journal of Clinical Psychiatry* (September 2004). http://www.ncbi.nlm.nih.gov/entrez/query.fcgi?cmd=Retrieve&db=pubmed&dopt=Abstract&list_uids=15367049.

Shenk, Joshua Wolf. "Lincoln's Great Depression." *Atlantic Monthly*, October 2005.

Stolberg, Sheryl Gay. "Preschool Meds." *The New York Times Magazine*, November 17, 2002.

Sugden, Stephen, and James Bourgeois. "Modafinil Monotherapy in Post-Stroke Depression." *Psychosomatics* (January–February 2004). http://repositories.cdlib.org/cgi/viewcontent.cgi?article=2727&context=postprints.

Trujillo, Keith, and Andrea Chin. "Antidepressants." *Drugs and the Brain*. California State University. http://www.csusm.edu/DandB/AD.html#history.

"US Epidemic: Controlled Prescription Drug Abuse—Teen Drug Abuse Triples in 10 Years." http://www.ahrp.org/infomail/05/07/09.php.

Watkins, Carol. "Seasonal Affective Disorder: Winter Depression." Northern County (Maryland) Psychiatric Associates (December 2004). http://www.ncpamd.com/seasonal.htm.

Wells, Kenneth B., Roland Sturm, and Cathy D. Sherbourne. *Caring for Depression*. Cambridge: Harvard University Press, 1996.

Windham, Christopher. "Ritalin Shows Promise in Treating Lethargy, Depression in Elderly." *Wall Street Journal*, July 17, 2003. http://ww2.aegis.org/news/wsj/2003/WJ030711.html.

"Wonder Drugs Misused: Teens Abusing and Selling Ritalin." http://www.campaignfortruth.com/Eclub/250303/wonderdrugmisused.htm.

Index

Picture Credits

iStockphotos: pp. 36, 39, 49, 73
   Anita Patterson: p. 70
   Chris Brantley: p. 69
   Chuck Spidell: p. 34
   Greg Nicholas: p. 66
   Jamie D. Travis: p. 29
   Joseph Jean Rolland Dubé: p. 31
   Karina Tischlinger: p. 96
   Kenneth C. Zirkel: p. 78
   Lisa F. Young: p. 56
   Marck Gucwa: p. 25
   Max Blain: p. 76
   Michael Knight: p. 50
   Nancy Louie: p. 26
   Piotr Przeszlo: p. 50
   Randall Schwanke: p. 33
   Suzanne Tucker: p. 83
   Tammy McAllister: p. 65
   Tom Boehler: p. 74
Jupiter Images: pp. 16, 19, 20, 52, 55, 58, 60, 80, 84, 87, 91, 93, 94
Library of Congress: pp. 9, 11
National Library of Medicine: pp. 22, 42

Biographies

Author

Craig Russell teaches writing at Broome Community College in Binghamton, New York. He has written several nonfiction books for young adults.

Consultant

Andrew M. Kleiman, M.D., received a Bachelor of Arts degree in philosophy from the University of Michigan, and earned his medical degree from Tulane University School of Medicine. Dr. Kleiman completed his internship, residency in psychiatry, and fellowship in forensic psychiatry at New York University and Bellevue Hospital. He is currently in private practice in Manhattan, specializing in psychopharmacology, psychotherapy, and forensic psychiatry. He also teaches clinical psychology at the New York University School of Medicine.